The Nurse Expert
Vol. 2

How to use radio to position yourself as the authority in your field

- A tool that every entrepreneurial nurse needs to be successful!

- Want to establish yourself as an expert? Radio is where it's at, and this book will help you successfully navigate your way to the top!

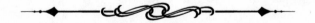

Dwayne Adams, RN, MS

www.TheNurseExpert.com
www.PRHealthCareCommunications.com

ISBN 978-0-9850033-0-2

Dedication

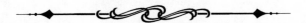

This book is dedicated to all of those in the field of nursing who are dedicated to helping others reach their health and wellness goals. Being a nurse shows just how much compassion, care and concern one has for others. Becoming an RN Health Coach further exemplifies that sense of dedication to helping others.

This book is dedicated to all nurses who have dedicated their lives to helping others, and to all those looking to further their career by becoming a successful health and wellness coach. I would also like to dedicate this book to the patients, who give us the opportunity to work with them in a coaching capacity as they strive to make important health improvements.

Finally, I would like to dedicate this book to my beautiful daughter, Aniyah, who continuously inspires me, and to all those who have helped in some way to develop my business, including graphic artists, writers and programmers. I couldn't have done it without all of you!

"Life's most urgent question is: what are you doing for others?" -- Martin Luther King, Jr.

Contents

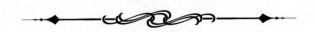

Preface

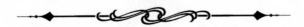

Over the past decade, I have had the privilege of working with a diverse population of nurses and other individuals in the healthcare field. Throughout those years, I have learned a great deal about nursing, but I have also spent time becoming a business-savvy entrepreneur.

Educated in both nursing and business, I have had an opportunity to learn what it takes to become a successful entrepreneur. I have studied and become an expert in the areas of marketing and sales, and I know what it takes to build, promote and sustain a successful business in the healthcare sector.

Through all of this, my own ideas on how to help others in nursing to capitalize on their skills and education have become an important priority. This book is the result of my ideas and my passion for helping other nurses to harness the power of their own skills and apply them to radio marketing opportunities.

Nurses should look to this book as a resourceful tool that will help enable them to become successful entrepreneurs in the health, wellness or nursing arenas.

Introduction

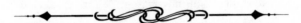

Welcome to "The Nurse Expert, Volume 2: How to Use Radio to Position Yourself as the Authority in Your Field." First, allow me to offer congratulations to you on taking this important step in furthering your career. The more you learn about how to be a successful entrepreneur and how to showcase your talents, skills and education, the better position you will be in. That's what this book aims to do – help you further your position and become a more successful entrepreneur in the area of providing health and wellness coaching or any other service you may provide as an entrepreneurial nurse.

With your specialized knowledge in health, you are in a prime position to become a successful entrepreneur. You have the skills and education that people need in order to reach their goals. Once you implement the ideas and advice set forth in this book, you will become more successful in your field.

This book is a tool that will help empower nurses to get away from the bedside and become actively involved in helping people to reach their health and wellness goals.

The pages that follow offer practical advice that is easy to follow and guaranteed to help ensure your success. Just think about how much radio is a part of your life. The same is true for the majority of people! Millions of individuals listen to the radio every week, and millions more are now listening to online radio, making it an important market for you to access.

By reading this book, you will learn why radio is a crucial medium that you should tap into, and how to successfully go about doing that. After reading this, you will become an authority on using radio in your area of expertise. Once your recognized as The Expert, you will be able to sell anything with ease. This book will give you the tools and tips you need in order to succeed!

As part of a series, this book is one of several that will help get you where you want to be. Covering radio is an important area, but it is not the only area you will want to skillfully master. Be sure to check out the other volumes in order to gain all the benefits you can, and to reach new levels in your coaching career!

Radio as a Free Marketing Tool

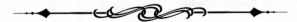

You have worked hard to establish yourself as a proficient and caring professional nurse. Without a doubt, you can reach the highest level of success in your private practice. But while you may have many people who know you and the work you do, it is imperative that you spread the word to as many people as possible by promoting your services when and wherever possible. Are you concerned that you may not be able to afford productive advertising at this stage in your career? That's where the services of my company come in.

My media outreach and public relations services will promote every aspect of your business, including your unique nursing services and professional accreditations. Radio can be used to promote your vast nursing experience and let your audience know how your practice is based upon this experience. Do you have a specific nursing expertise? Promote your specialty and your overall nursing skills so that listeners can understand that you are a well rounded nursing professional.

In this chapter, we will begin to cover the building blocks of successful radio marketing. I will outline the reasons behind its success, which will provide you with some points to think about if you are making a decision whether to utilize this marketing tool. The related subjects in this chapter are:

-**What can we promote?** Jump start your creativity by reading about some potential promotion ideas.

-**The Power of Radio.** Does this media option really have the ability to help market your business?

-**The Media Needs You.** Get insider information on why radio stations need you.

-**Paid Advertising vs. Press Coverage.** Weighing in on the pros and cons of each of these options based on these factors:

- Cost
- Audience attention
- The trust factor
- Increased exposure

What can we promote?

Utilizing free radio as a marketing tool also provides a chance for you to promote your website and relay important contact information to a wide audience at one time. Promote your past and present success stories via radio marketing, and at the same time listeners will get an idea of your personality and "bedside manner" and the vision you have for your practice into the future.

Believe it or not, free radio advertising can jump start your practice very quickly. As a health and wellness expert, I am able to effectively establish your presence in the industry using this very effective, free media source. My business has successfully coached Registered Nurses in many specialty areas. I have developed a popular, comprehensive nursing opportunity program that opens the opportunity for nurses to learn how to build their own health coach practice, which is quickly becoming one of the fastest growing health care fields. The program takes the nurse through each step in the process to build the rewarding, successful practice they dream of. Details of this exciting program opportunity can be found at **RNHealthCoach.com or HealthCoachNursingJobs.com.**

The Power of Radio

You would be surprised how much radio advertising can rapidly catapult your dreams into reality. Throughout the decades, authors, entertainers, entrepreneurs and many others have used this media to get the word out about themselves and precisely what they do. Millions of people who listen to the radio have been convinced, with just one interview, that they simply must have the service or product they heard about on the radio.

Think about it, how many times have you been driving in the car and heard a commercial jingle for a certain product that stayed in your mind all day? Most likely, you or the millions of other people who heard the commercial bought that widget, gadget or service connected to the jingle. Have you ever wondered how much the company paid for the airtime to advertise their product? In almost every instance, the company paid nothing; it simply took advantage of free radio advertising offered by radio stations across the nations. It is estimated that more than 10,000 of these opportunities are available each and every day.

For instance, the authors of "Chicken Soup for the Soul" have enjoyed well over a staggering 100 million in book sales. They were asked what they believed was the secret to such phenomenal success. Would you believe they credited telephone interviews with radio stations as the number one reason that their books flew off the shelves? Yes, they reported that they participated in at least one interview each day at radio stations across the country. As you know, this strategy paid off immensely.

Strategic, professional publicity and marketing by means of radio has been the key to success for countless others including best selling author M. Scot Peck (The Road Less Traveled), Earl Mindell (Vitamin Bible) and many others. Without exception, these successful people have utilized radio interviews, which have greatly contributed to their great achievements.

I can help guide you in the promotion of your own practice by teaching you how to present yourself on the radio as an expert on the subject. I will show you how to have the confidence to speak with authority about the nursing profession, your role and the unique services that you offer. Why shell out millions of dollars to promote your nursing practice when I can help you join others who have taken advantage of free radio advertising with fantastic results?

How does utilizing free radio marketing translate into advertising dollars savings and profitability? One author reports that he promoted his successful book almost exclusively through radio interviews. He estimates that he participated in over 1300 hundred interviews that aired on over 2,700 radio stations. The result? The interviews helped to generate over one and a half million dollars in sales! And what would be the approximate cost for advertising that would generate this amount? It would have cost the author a whopping five million dollars to pay for such promotion- and he shelled out no money whatsoever!

The lesson for you, the budding private nurse practice owner, is that the more exposure you get, the more profit you can expect. And those profits can be even larger with free radio advertising.

The Media Needs You

Most likely, by now you have many questions about how free radio marketing works. In addition, you may be skeptical because you are unsure why a radio station would want to give you, a professional nurse, free advertising for your private practice. In order to understand how the process works, the first thing you need to know is that the media not only wants you, but they need you. Think about the last time a really interesting television reality show caught your attention. Most likely, it held your attention because it was entertaining, yet it combined real life situations that you could either learn from or relate to. The media knows this is a winning combination, and this is the basis of how free radio advertising works.

I will use my expertise to show you how to use knowledge about the media to your own advantage. For instance, the media is well aware that people make the best sources for programming. Their goal is to not only entertain the audience, but to enlighten and inform their listening public. As a nurse, you represent the cream of the crop when it comes to filling the media's needs. Your own unique style, combined with intelligence, makes an interview with you very entertaining. Combine this with the wealth of information that you can share with the public regarding health care, nursing and your private practice, and it is no wonder that any radio station would be glad to air your story.

Here's how it works: The media makes money from selling advertising. It is very important that they maintain high ratings in order to be able to demand the highest premium possible for advertising on their station. If ratings show a decrease in listeners, the advertising revenues of the station are also reduced. As such, the media will go out of their way to attract as many listeners as possible. This is accomplished by providing <u>interesting, entertaining and informative programming</u>. Please don't forget this winning combo of a formula. Together with my PR services designed just for nurses, we will design such a show.

As a professional nurse, you can offer your wide range of skills, including interesting stories and observations relating to your career. Similar to a barter system, the media is all too happy to accept the terrific programming you provide in exchange for letting you share information about your practice. My promotion services will groom you so that you can present yourself as a nursing professional while at the same time keep the listening audience interested in what you have to say. I employ public relations strategies that will equip you to present yourself effectively and promote your business in a manner that will put you on the short list for radio interviews all over the country.

But make no mistake, it takes planning in order to create the right package that will prove to the media that you are a valuable guest that will keep people listening. I am an expert in health care public relations. Visit my websites at www.PRHealthCareCommunications.com or **www. MedicalMarketingSEO.com** to find out how I can promote your nursing practice by putting it in the best light with the finest website design and Search Engine Optimization services available.

Paid Advertising vs. Press Coverage

If you're still reading, you are probably weighing your options for promoting your nursing practice. You may be considering paying for advertising, or at the very least wondering whether press coverage is to your true advantage as compared to paying for advertising. Naturally, you want to present your practice to the public in an organized and professional manner. You may be hesitant to investigate free radio marketing because you are concerned about the quality of no cost advertising. On the other hand, perhaps your advertising budget prohibits you from advertising; which could be costing you even more money.

You are not the first nurse who has faced this dilemma when opening his or her own practice, which is why I am here to help. It is not my job to set you up for failure; rather, I am committed to promoting your practice in ways that will result in ultimate success.

I am confident in my services, especially since I have developed several nurse coaching programs that have proven to be successful for RN's in private practice in many nursing specialties. The umbrella company, L.I.T.E. Therapeutics, Inc, is a fully comprehensive support system for private practice nurses with coaching specialties that include weight loss, disease management, smoking cessation and corporate wellness. I specialize in helping nurses to create and maintain very lucrative business opportunities, despite dismal employment statistics. And I don't stop there-I will guide you through the marketing and promotion process that is a key element to the success of your business.

In order to help you make the right decision, let's compare paid marketing and promotion with publicity resulting from promotion as a radio show guest.

-Cost. The price for advertising can be tens of thousands of dollars for 60 seconds of advertising, depending on the station. As we have already covered, the cost to be interviewed on a radio station is free. You can promote your nursing practice at no cost, as long as you find an interesting "hook", leaving money for other improvements and expenditures. See *The Nurse Expert Vol. 1*, for details on creating that winning hook that is needed.

-Audience attention. It is a fact that people pay more attention to the show they are watching or listening to than the commercials. For instance, how many times have you gotten up for a glass of water during a commercial, or channel surfed while a commercial was on the radio? The same applies to paid radio advertising; listeners are much more likely to stay tuned to the actual show (on which you will promote your practice) than stick around and wait to hear a commercial.

-The trust factor. It is just human nature for people to be skeptical about what they hear in a commercial. Many people are distrustful of outright "sales tactics". The majority of listeners believe that media reports, such as interviews and stories, are unbiased. Whether or not this is a fact is not important. What is important is that I can help you to use the tendency that people have to trust content more than advertising to your advantage when promoting your nursing practice on the radio.

-Increased exposure. A medium sized radio station has about 3,000 listeners each second. Large stations have 30,000 people listening in every second of the day. This is one of the reasons why many entrepreneurs like you choose to learn how to capitalize on the millions of people who tune in to radio interviews every week. And unlike the common commercial that crams in information in sixty seconds at a very fast pace, a radio interview will allow you to take more time to give a thorough presentation about your nursing service(s).

So, even if you are lucky enough to have millions of dollars to spend on advertising, why pay such an expense when you can get equal, and often better, results for free? As a new nursing practice owner, most likely you do not have the advertising budget of large corporations, many of whom pay over $500 for each minute of advertising. Alternatively, you can get more than $12,000 worth of free advertising, without rushing through a 60-second commercial spot. Statistics report that well over 200 million people listen to the radio in a week. Why not capture your share of those listeners and save big bucks for your practice at the same tThese are just a few comparisons of the advantages of radio interviews verses paid on-air advertising. I am committed to helping promote your nursing practice to as wide an audience as possible. I have done the math for you and am happy to share my research efforts with you to save you time and money while presenting your practice in the best light possible.

Radio as the Superior Medium

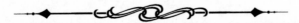

In this chapter, we will delve into the details of exactly why radio promotion is the better choice for advertising. Our research has uncovered numerous reasons why a nursing professional should choose this form of promotion. My company will be very pleased to represent your best interests every step of the way, so you never have to be concerned that your publicity is not reflecting your business according to your specifications.

This chapter will cover issues such as how plugging your business is the quickest way to see profits, and why radio marketing is the superior avenue to choose. Increasing the numbers in your target audience, very important to success, is also covered in this chapter. You will learn how radio marketing adds even more money to your bottom line in terms of travel and other expenses.

In order to provide you with all the information needed to reach the goals for your business, I will cover areas such as appearance, shyness, fear and other matters that affect your business. My goal is to keep you well informed about the reasons why I believe that my services can be one of the essential tools used to help you reach ultimate success in your business.

Profit from Plugs

In the first chapter, I discussed the basics of how free radio publicity works. As you know, publicity comes in many forms; the two ways that people broadcast their businesses, products and services are radio and television. As covered in the previous chapter, radio publicity can be in the form of paid advertising or free radio marketing. The same goes for television. However, radio proves to be clearly superior over television for marketing purposes for several reasons.

In order for people to purchase a product or contract a service, they need to know how to contact the business. As a nursing coach, you will want people to know where to go to find more information, such as your website. Or you may have a toll free number that people can call, which you will want to provide to listeners.

Relating this information at the interview has often been jokingly referred to as a "shameless plug", which means the interviewee is not trying to hide the fact that he or she is soliciting business. Actually, this plug can mean serious profits, so it is important that this information be relayed clearly before the interview ends. In fact, you should expect an almost immediate reaction once you have provided listeners with the contact information for your business.

However, while the majority of radio stations gladly allow their program guests to plug their books, movies, products or services in exchange for entertaining and informational program content, most television programs do not allow this practice. The rationale behind this refusal is that viewers will assume that the station is endorsing the business, which most are certainly not willing to do.

Larger Audience for Your Message

I have compiled some statistics for you that will bring home this point. Don't assume, as most people do, that radio has been replaced entirely by television and the Internet. I have carefully researched the patterns of radio listeners in order to provide effective assistance for your marketing needs. As such, I have uncovered some very interesting statistics about radio listeners.

-**Number of stations.** There is a vastly larger radio audience than has long been assumed. On average, these 75 percent of weekly radio listeners tune in to six stations each week. They tend to tune in for several short bursts, probably switching during commercials as we discussed on the first chapter.

-Higher number of listeners. While it has been reported that about 73 percent of people older than 12 years listen to the radio daily, recent data reports that the number is closer to 85 percent. That's a huge listening audience that I can help you to tap into to generate interest in your business.

-Time of day. Further data points to evidence that the time of day these radio listeners tune in is scattered throughout the day. Therefore, you can expect that listeners, which include early morning commuters, employees on lunch break as well as night shift workers, will be among the people who will hear about your nursing practice throughout the day.

For these and many other reasons, radio is the clear choice for free advertising that will reach the greatest number of people. Let me utilize my years of experience, research and resources to help you promote your nursing practice as effectively as possible in the shortest amount of time.

Travel Savings

Contrary to popular belief, it is far from glamorous to travel from city to city doing television interviews. Naturally, you are expected to travel to the television studio itself or perhaps an affiliate studio in which satellite interviews can be taped. Without exception, you will encounter more than your fair share of mishaps, hassles and other travel related issues. Letting me help you market your business by means of radio interviews will solve the majority of these headaches. You will have the stress free ease of staying at your own home to do the interview. I can't tell you how many of my nursing coach business clients have expressed the sheer luxury and convenience of interviewing from home, sometimes from the comfort of their own bed.

In addition to saving money for travel expenses, you keep money in your pocket for long distance phone charges because, without exception, it will be the radio station that calls you for the interview. With the help of my marketing and promotion services (see www. PRHealthCareCommunications.com), you too can be heard by the captive audiences who are in their cars, at home or on their job.

There are many other advantages to marketing your business through free radio promotion. One of these advantages is being able to do your business promotion from absolutely anywhere on the planet. I will show you how to arrange radio interviews, regardless of where you live, with radio stations around the world. Since this is already being done by millions of people from other countries who wish to promote their products and services in America, why don't you let me help you to market your business to other English speaking radio stations in other countries? I can help you get the word out regardless of where the station is located, and regardless of what location you may be in at any given time.

Appearance Doesn't Count

As a nursing coach professional, you know all too well that how you look can make or break your business while you are in the presence of your clients. Imagine how much more important your appearance becomes when you are in front of television cameras that are broadcasting your image to millions of people. You would never take a chance on not presenting the best possible image to the public. You are the first impression that people get of your business. Therefore, in order to put your best foot forward, you would most likely spend money to hire a stylist, which could be quite expensive, especially if you are slated to give several interviews.

This is another reason why radio marketing is the superior choice for promoting your nursing practice. You will not have to worry about how you look during the interview because you will, in this case, be heard and not seen. This strategy also saves you money in wardrobe costs, since you will need a different set of clothes for each television interview. Radio marketing is also a solution for people who are working through confidence issues regarding their appearance.

Elimination of Public Fear

Not everyone is comfortable speaking in public. This condition, also known as performance anxiety or stage fright, is reportedly the number one fear in adults. By some estimates, 90 percent of adults have a fear of speaking in public to some degree. Moreover, while getting the word out about your business is absolutely critical, this fear can inhibit some people to the point that it does damage to their business image.

If you suffer with performance anxiety, I will help to market your business on the radio, which can be less stressful for you. Without the thought of millions of people staring at you and critiquing your every move, you will be able to express your thoughts and share your business in a much more effective manner. Countless business owners, authors, celebrities and others have used radio media to promote themselves with equal or greater success than television interviews. Radio promotion is a means for you to generate direct business while working toward transitioning to more visual media, such as television, to market your business. This is another reason that radio marketing is a far better choice to publicize your business.

Four Ways to Get on the Radio as an Expert

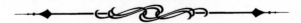

As you can see, radio interviews can be used to promote you and your nursing coach business. But, as you can guess, it takes some effort to secure radio interviews. There are several ways to find radio stations seeking people to interview. However, each comes with its good and not so good points. I will incorporate my marketing and public relations experience to navigate the waters for you.

I have included the following helpful topics in this chapter to help you get you started.

- Pitch to producers via mail, fax or email

- Advertise in directories

- Hire a PR Firm

- Contact and pitch directly to producers

Pitch to producers via mail, fax or email

It is possible to get a booking for a radio interview by introducing yourself and your business to radio producers, but only if they are able to hear what you have to offer. Providing producers with information about your business is known as "pitching", and it is very tricky and requires careful planning and correct choices of format. I hope that you have read The

Nurse Expert, Vol 1, as it provides just the information you need to do this. I can help you increase your chances of being booked because I understand what producers are looking for with guests for their programs. Naturally, radio producers are very particular about how their guests sound to the audience since radio is an auditory media. Unless your pitch is as near perfect as possible, there is no chance you will be invited to be a guest on the show. And truthfully, this simply cannot be accomplished by the producers simply reading your promotional materials. Of course, with good writing you can give producers somewhat of an idea of the topic you may cover during an interview. However, the written information cannot convey the tone and sound of your voice, your personality, or your ability to keep the audience listening. Therefore, sending an informational pamphlet in the mail is quite useless in getting booked for radio interviews. There are ways I can combine your written promotional material with media to give producers a more comprehensive preview, which I will discuss later in the chapter.

But what about contacting radio station program producers using email? Again, this is not an effective way of getting the true essence of you and your business into the hands of radio show producers. Even if you attach audio (and/or video) to your email, it will most likely not produce the results you expect basically for two reasons:

1. **It may never be seen.** You can only imagine how much email producers receive every day. It's a good guess that the majority of these are never opened, are deleted by the producer's staff, or end up in the spam folder and are then automatically deleted. Therefore, the chances that your email will be opened are very slim.

2. **Quality.** Let's say by some chance that your email did catch the attention of the producer and he decides to open it. For any number of reasons, the quality of the attachment could be compromised or the audio or video files may improperly download. Why take chances when this could be your only possible shot at pitching your business to this producer?

A word of caution about email lists. There are many companies on the Internet that will try to convince you to pay money for a list of contact information for radio and other media producers. These lists are not cheap, yet many people have spent a lot of money for lists that contain a lot of contact information which prove useless. It does not help you to have contact information for stations that are too remote or tiny to serve any real purpose. This means that, although you may get their attention, it is not worth your effort to follow through. Or, again, the list could send you down the unproductive path of sending out emails to larger stations in vain. Let my experience in marketing and promotions help you to weed out any options that will prove to be a waste of time and money. Avoid stations with less than 10,000 listeners. It's just not worth your time!

The same theories hold true for sending unsolicited faxes to pitch your business. Most everyone resents uninvited contact in any form. But large radio stations especially dislike the interruption and invasiveness of fax blasts, so it is best used sparingly, if at all. A lot of new business owners employ the strategy of sending faxes to stations on their email lists whenever a news story breaks that relates to their industry. They include an interesting point of view that might pique the interest of the producer, and then follow up with a quick phone call. Sometimes if the topic is a hot subject that is currently in the news, this effort can result in a request for an interview. Again, reaching out to producers through regular mail, email or faxes should be approached with caution combined with a well-planned strategy.

Advertise in Directories

You are not alone in having limited advertising resources as a new business owner. However, you can still effectively promote your business on a low budget by advertising in directories specifically designed to showcase up and coming businesses and talent. These directories are available in every major city, nationally and in every country in the world. They can be found in trade magazines, telephone directories and on the Internet. You too can join millions of others to draw the attention of radio producers using this medium.

One successful network, The Association of Independents in Radio (AIR), is comprised of over 800 radio media, television and other producers. The organization functions as a primary advocate for commercial and public media producers. On their website, AIR has a talent directory available for members to list their information. While most people in the directory are seeking positions in radio or television as artists, producers or news reporters, it can also be a good avenue to post your business information since there is a good chance it will be seen by radio producers.

Another popular directory can be found in the magazine RTIR (Radio Television Interview Report), which more accurately targets individuals and businesses that seek to get free radio publicity by becoming a guest on radio or television programs. According to their website, the magazine is viewed by more than 4,000 media producers seeking suitable guests for their programs. The magazine staff will help to prepare your pitch and place it in the magazine at a very reasonable cost. RTIR has received high praise for their contribution to the success in helping people garner interest for radio interviews. Ad promotion in this magazine has resulted in almost immediate responses and in many cases, has led to radio interviews that have ended with increased exposure and profits for the business owners.

Hire a PR Firm

Another option for promoting your business is to hire a public relations firm. If you chose this option, be prepared to pay a premium for their services. Most public relations firms will require an up-front, non-refundable retainer fee. There is no guarantee that the firm will acquire interviews for you. A good public relations firm will charge, at a minimum, a couple thousand dollars a month. Larger firms can cost $10,000 per month. My PR firm is solely for the RN with a budget in mind.

You have heard of the adage, "you get what you pay for". This especially applies to public relations contracting. If a firm offers to work for you for a very low price, you can be pretty sure you will get the worst offers possible, if those. Offers from radio stations that are too small, too remote or do their interviews during unfavorable time slots equate to no interviews at all since no one is likely to hear your interview anyway. I am in no way implying that it is not possible to hire a good public relations firm. However, in order to see the best results you should be prepared to pay a cost. As it relates to hiring a public relations firm, there are a few key areas to watch for and to be very cautious of. These areas are top markets, wattage and pricing.

-**Top markets don't mean a lot.** One public relations trick that so many new businesses fall for is when the firm sells them on the idea that they will only book them on the "top market" shows. They inflate the importance of these so-called top markets by telling you they are the 100, 25 or 10 so called top markets. In actuality, this does not mean anything when it comes to promoting your business. How markets work is this: In America, the number one market is the city of New York. So in theory, all radio stations with transmitters can claim that they have a number one market ranking, just based on the fact that they are broadcasting from the city. But the catch is that this means that all radio stations, from the largest to the smallest unknown station, can actually be said to have number one ranking.

With this scenario, which is repeated all over the country, you can risk paying thousands of dollars for a highly rated radio station, when the station only has the rating because they happen to be in a metropolitan area that is top rated. I do not want you to give up on radio advertising because you did not get a response after doing interviews with a so-called number one rated radio station. It could be that the public relations market led you to believe that top market rankings were equivalent to a large number of listeners, but in many cases, this is not necessarily the case.

-**Wattage can be meaningless.** Be cautious if a public relation firm tries to sell you on stations based upon their wattage alone. Some will tell you that they will book you exclusively with stations that have a higher wattage of up 50,000 or more. Since you are new to the industry, you may mistakenly believe that this automatically means that you will become very popular overnight. But allow me to explain what this can really mean in terms of promotion for your business. In a nutshell, higher wattage is usually found in the smaller, not larger, radio stations. This is because in bigger cities there are large numbers of stations competing for listeners. You have experienced this when driving through big cities and finding stations at every stop along the dial. Therefore, the FCC must reduce the wattage on the transmitters of all of those radio stations. If not, the signals of the large number of radio stations would bleed and interfere with one another; thus, making it hard for listeners to tune in to any station at all.

Can you remember the last time you were listening to the radio in a remote location? Most likely, you were able to tune in to a couple of stations that came in loud and clear. This is because, in response to the issue mentioned above, the FCC doles out loads of wattage to radio stations with low population. Again, the wattage that a station has is proportionate to the number of listeners in the area. The smaller the area, the more wattage is given by the FCC, and vise versa. It is important that you not allow yourself to be taken advantage of by a firm that charges you a lot of money for bookings with high wattage. Not many new business owners seeking to promote themselves on the radio are aware of this. I am able to share my past experience with you to help you avoid such mistakes.

Investigating price philosophy of PR firms. I want to stress to you, use these suggestions upon hiring a PR firm. They include:

- Always compare agencies in order to get a general idea what a firm should charge for various services. Even though you may be quoted an hourly rate, many firms add a price for specific projects or tasks.

- Establish a budget that is reasonable for you. Give the firm an idea of what it is you expect them to accomplish and ask that they give specific fees for the services you require. A good public relations firm will not balk at providing you with precise quotes for their work, including hourly rates and creative fees.

- When you are comparing firms, compare the costs for all types of public relations including freelance, in-house teams and agencies. This will give you a wider range to compare since each of these types charge differently.

- As with any industry, public relation firms have their share of both good and not-so-good providers. If you are interested in a certain agency, get as many references as possible and follow through with contacting those references. Word of mouth, whether positive or negative, can help you make a better choice than going it alone.

Contact and Pitch Directly to Producers

By far, the most effective way to get radio interviews is by direct contact to the producers of the big stations. My media and marketing business, PR Health Care Communications, prides itself on being able to get your pitch into the hands of the people who count. I have a complete database of the highest rated radio shows, and I know how to maximize use of this database in order to get results for you very quickly. All that you need to make the right impression, including a website optimized to reel in interested producers, will be included in my services. I have vast experience in speaking with producers in their own language, so to speak, to represent you as the competent, exciting and interested expert that radio stations are looking to interview.

The Two Essential Tools Needed

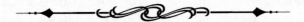

By now, I'm sure you are excited about the prospect of promoting your business by means of radio marketing. As I've outlined, there are big advantages to using this absolutely free tool to people who are looking for nursing coaches who are experts in their field. But before you even begin to contact radio show producers there are some essential things you will need. One of the main tools that you must have is a database of the high-ranking radio shows, which includes contact information. This list must be current in order to do the job it is intended to do, which is to reach out to the producers in order to pitch your business. The other essential tool is a top notch, absolutely spectacular press kit. In this chapter, I will give you, in detail, the information you need to fulfill these two important needs.

Database of the Top Radio Shows

Without this tool, it is impossible to reach the people you need to get you on the air. But before I begin, I would like to emphasize that this list MUST be current and include contacts. Too much time and money has been wasted purchasing old, inaccurate or incomplete databases. This is another area in which my marketing and public relations firm can be of help to you. I maintain a comprehensive and exhaustive list of top ranking shows. My list not only provides contact information and station locations, but completely accurate listener numbers for each station. Unfortunately, many new businesses have purchased so-called databases that are blatantly inaccurate; some even include listener numbers higher than the entire population of the city in which the station does business.

So don't be fooled by statistic reports that even ten percent radio listeners in a location is considered as good numbers. But again, I have done the work for you and will be able to access only the most accurate databases for you.

I do not put "fillers" in the database, which means I do not include talk stations that have less than 100,000 listeners. Contact information, including email addresses, for the host and the producers are included in my database. I include the names of the News and Program Directors as well as the Public Affairs Directors. I describe each talk show and include biographies of the hosts and what kinds of guests they are looking for. This is very helpful to you in order to prepare to pitch your business. As a nursing coach, you want to make sure you're not wasting time pitching to a show that is only interested in guests who are in a specific unrelated field. Since it has been proven that shows that run through the night or before sunrise on weekends get very few listeners, I do not include these stations in the database.

In order to provide precise, useful information, I list each and every market that the station reaches. I include nearby cities so that you get a better idea of how many people will be tuning in to your interview. The website addresses, which can include very helpful information, are also among the information included in my database. I even provide time zones for the stations so you will know the best times to call.

My database is sorted by category, making it quicker and easier to sort. Among the categories is health, which is naturally of interest to you. In addition, radio shows relating to travel, legal, food, general interest, psychology and many more categories are included. You would be surprised at how many of these other categories are interested in interviewing someone like you, since your nurse coaching is related to many fields. I think outside of the box, and include station information for talk shows on topics such as metaphysics, spiritual issues and empowerment. While these talk shows may not get as many listeners as others, I have included them in a specialized database; their targeted and precise topics can also draw interest in your nursing coaching. And most importantly, I keep the database fresh and current with updates.

Press Kit

Our medical marketing services will provide you with a brilliant, search engine optimized website, which will go a long way towards promoting your business. However, you will still need a hard copy of all of the information about your business in the form of a press kit. Nothing is as important as having the most comprehensive, eye-catching press kit you possibly can. Without this, phone calls, websites and other means are quite useless to the radio station and here's why:

- A huge part of your image is your ability to stand out from the crowd. You might be surprised at how many newer business owners rely solely on their websites as the means to get their brand or image across. Therefore, it stands to reason that the moment a radio station lays eyes on your fabulous press kit that it will make a good impression. It will convey the image that you are not only serious about yourself and your business, but that you are willing to put your money where your mouth is and spend cash to put together a professional press kit. In many cases, this has been the key to getting preferential treatment and quick bookings.

- It takes just a quick second to click off of a webpage. However, if a personalized press kit is delivered to the station, many times it is hard for producers to just throw it in the trash. In many cases, the time and expense you have put into the press kit is enough for the producer to at least give it a good look. I will show you how to present the kit for mailing so that it gives the exact impression you are trying to convey.

- The physical, hard copy of a press kit is more likely to be brought to the table when producers sit around the table for brainstorming meetings. Having the press kit in hand is more convenient for the producer than having to print out your media page from your website. The press kit lends credibility to your business, which makes it easier for the producer to pitch you for an interview on the show.

For these and many other reasons, I strongly encourage you not to skimp on this most important marketing tool. Remember, it will grab the attention of the producer, which is the first step toward getting that interview. Include it as an addition to your media page on the website, which will give you a chance to give the producer options for getting your information. A good tactic is to tell the producer that you will send over a press kit, even if they don't ask. This lets them know you are serious about wanting a chance to be interviewed. Before we get into the precise details of what should be in your press kit, let's explore the exact purpose of the kit and what it is supposed to accomplish.

The purpose of a press kit is to first identify you, which is the reason that a biography is included. Who you are also includes credentials, which will be important to the producer. The press kit also lets the producer know what it is you intend to say to the audience. It will express the idea you have for the show. Your press kit should let the producer know that your idea will be of benefit to the audience in one or more ways. The kit will also include your contact information and finally, you will let the producer know just what it is that you are promoting. Your press kit should fully explain your services; maybe even include the cost or other details if you have time. This transparency will give the producer an idea if your interest conflicts with the stations' in any way.

Below are the basic elements of a press kit. Although there are several parts to the kit, some are more important than others are; such as, the pitch sheet and sample questions. Even so, the press sheet should be of quality from start to finish and presented in a professional manner.

-**Housing.** The press kit must be housed within a double pocket folder or portfolio. The housing should have a top quality matte finish; never glossy because it leaves fingerprints. Purchasing the folders in bulk is not only less expensive but more convenient to do. Again, never skimp on quality for your press kit housing.

-**Cover.** The outside of the press kit portfolio should have a photo, color graphic or even book cover. The purpose is to get immediate attention, but make sure it relates to your topic in some manner. For instance, you could have graphics that relate to weight loss or whatever your nursing coach specialty entails.

-Business card. All quality portfolios and folders come with a slot for business cards. Use this to place your dazzling professional (preferably color) business card. In most instances, it is the business card that the producer retains, sometimes long after other elements of the press kit have been discarded. Therefore, make sure that the card contains crucial information which make include your picture, all contact information including your website, your credentials and other necessities.

-Press release. The actual press release or the show pitch sheet is the most vital element of your press kit. It should be the very top sheet in the left side pocket of the portfolio. This is because by nature, people read from the left side to the right side, so the producer will look at the left side first. Make sure you maintain the utmost quality with your press release, including appearance, paper quality and content. The press release should be in full color and grab attention right away. Although you can create your own press release, whenever possible have it professionally done to avoid mistakes or the possibility of it looking cheap. Any price you pay will be well worth the effort. And remember, you are preparing to get thousands of dollars in free radio publicity, so the price will be well worth it.

Since this is the most important piece of paper in your press kit, let's go into detail how to prepare the most winning pitch sheet possible. In the furthermost top left corner, you should have the words "Available for Interview". This is called the identifier. You've seen identifiers in traditional press releases, commonly with the words "For Immediate Release". The same principle applies to you, you are letting the producer know that you are ready to be "released", or interviewed as a guest on their radio show. Oftentimes it is a good idea to emphasize the identifier with a gold sticker that can be imprinted with the words of the identifier.

Next to the identifier, you should have your contact information. The contact can be you or someone else, but the name, all phone numbers and email address should be in this section. Beneath the identifier and contact information, at the top of the press release, should be the headline. The headline should be one line in large bold letters that have big impact. It is the headline that is the powerful "hook" that grabs the producer, so compose it carefully. The feel of the headline is somewhat like an article in the newspaper that gives you a teaser of the interesting information to follow. Play around with different ideas for your headline that relates to your nursing practice. Have fun with it and get friends to help come up with jaw dropping headlines. Most headlines are about seven words, but can be a little longer but not too lengthy.

Your photo should be situated directly beneath your headline in the far right column at the top. Choose your photo carefully; making sure it is an image that portrays you at your best. As a nursing coach, you want to have a photo that represents your profession and shouts credibility and interest.

The photo specifications are:

- Color photograph
- Tight head shot
- Stops at the upper chest

The purpose of the photograph is to give the producer the chance to match the press release with the person it applies to. Some people put captions under the photos that state credentials and experience, but it is not necessary.

Very important to the press release is the **bullet box**. The bullet box is located to the far left under the headline. It is also known as a callout box. Some bullet boxes have borders to make them stand out. What makes them important is they contain bullet points of the key elements you will be presenting to the radio audience. This section must be carefully composed and edited. Do not make the mistake of putting too much information or writing dull uninteresting verbiage in the bullet box. Next to the headline, it must be the next thing that immediately jumps out and tells the producer exactly what you are going to say to the listeners in a concise manner. Pay careful attention to these bullet points and continue to work with them until they are precise and compelling. This takes knowing the highlights of what you do and teasing the producer to want to know too. Statistics related to your field also look good in bullet points and gives the producer something to consider.

Your **biography**, or bio, should be included in the press kit. It should briefly cover your identify, credentials, career experience and any other radio or television interviews you have done on the subject. The bio is positioned in the far right corner of the press release, directly under your photograph.

Be sure to include your **contact information** under the press release, even though it is included on your business card. Most press releases put this information in a border that spans the same width as the headline. You may also request a CD of the interview, if they are chosen for the program.

Sample questions should be placed directly behind the press release (left pocket). Make sure that you list no more than 15 sample interview questions on one page only. Take time to choreograph this carefully in order to be fully prepared for the interview. The host and producer will be pleased that you have provided these questions because it will save them time. Most likely, they will ask the questions exactly as you have written them with few changes. There are times, however, when a host will throw in a trick question. Do not take it personally, but prepare yourself to remain as calm as possible in the event this happens. Sample questions can include the reason you went into nursing, coaching and the specialty you've chosen. You may initially want to answer questions about why you consider yourself an expert in order to establish your credentials. A simple way to think of questions is to pull from the points in your bullet box. Your sample questions should provide the producer with the approximate time it will take to ask and answer them. This will help immensely in planning the show. If, by some chance, your coaching has an element of controversy, you will inform the producer by preparing a controversy sheet, although it is not required.

If you prefer, you can include a cover letter in your press kit. It should be placed as the very first sheet in the right pocket of the portfolio. Basically, the cover letter reiterates the press release, and it has been my experience that producers don't usually read them. If you chose to compose a cover letter, it should outline the topic in the first four lines. The next paragraph should explain how your topic will interest their audience or provide them with information. The following lines should be a step-by-step list of what you plan to say to the office with emphasis on the content, not solicitation of your services. Following this is a small biographical paragraph and lastly, any radio or television interviews, then a convincing line or two about why you should be chosen for an interview. The cover letter is not a required element of your press kit. Another option is to put a little hand written note in the press release to thank them for their time and to express enthusiasm that you will hear from them. A small reminder of the gist of your conversation with the producer can be a nice touch too.

If you use a cover letter, the next pieces in the right hand pocket are any testimonials or clippings you may have. If your business has been reviewed in magazines or newspapers, include these clippings to impress the producer. Add any letters from other show hosts or producers to show that you have successfully handled interviews before, if applicable. Make sure that this documentation is less than six months old.

If any of your clients have written letters of thanks or testimonials about your services, including success stories, they should be among this group of documents. If you are booked for an interview, don't forget to politely ask for a testimonial or written feedback that you can add to your press kit for the next potential interview. Although you may believe that producers will think negatively about this strategy, in actuality it will open more doors for you. Think of how much more willing you are to purchase a product or service if you hear from someone else how satisfied they were with their purchase. In the same way, a testimony can serve somewhat as a reference for you.

As they say, "the devil is in the details". Even the professional and stunning press kit can be ruined if it is mailed in an inappropriate envelope. Don't leave out this important detail; make it as impressive as the press kit itself. Again, you want to stand out from the crowd of other kits on the producer's desk, so make the envelope count. The envelope must be 10" x 13" to accommodate the portfolio. Envelopes in these sizes come in all kinds of vibrant colors; try to coordinate it with the colors within the press kit. The manner in which you address the envelope will also say a lot about your professionalism. Mailing labels should not be used. Rather, it should be neatly hand printed to provide a personal touch, perhaps with a thick permanent marker that will be sure to get attention. You will not send a press kit unless it is requested, so you should print the words "*material requested enclosed*", or similar on the envelope. This statement will also avoid interns or secretaries from throwing out the press kit since they can see the producer requested it.

Keys to Finding the Right Shows

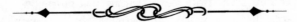

Now that you've gotten an idea of how radio marketing can promote your business and learned more about public relations firms, press releases and other matters it is time to target the shows that should be contacted. This is another service that my marketing and promotions company can offer to you. Sorting through the various kinds of radio station shows can be confusing since there are so many types. News and music stations, shock-jocks, FM talk shows and syndication all have shows that include interviewing guests.

However, it is important that you target the shows that are compatible with your nursing business. Why is this important? For one thing, you do not want to risk damaging your reputation by being known for accepting just any interview for the publicity. Secondly, your time and effort are very valuable. You do not have the luxury of wasting either or both of these by interviewing on shows that will not help in the promotion of your business. Nevertheless, you must now develop a system of how and who to call once you have found the right shows.

It is at this point that the database we discussed becomes your lifeline. In fact, you will not know whom to call without having access to my comprehensive database. The process of combing the database should be as follows:

- Start by reading through the description of shows and make a mark next to all of the possible shows that apply to your nurse business.

- During the above step, eliminate only the shows that have absolutely no relation to your business. For instance, a show about "bowling" will not relate to your nursing career. However, don't be too hasty. If there is a topic that may apply to nursing, do not eliminate it. For example, a show titled "Healthy Food" can be tied in to your weight loss nursing program; even though the title does not include weight loss or nursing.

- Categorize and use a separate mark for the shows that directly target your niche from those that are just possibilities. This way you can distinguish the more desirable shows at a quick glance, which will save you time.

- Starting with the target shows, sort the shows by time. Shows that air in the morning will be the first that you pitch because more people listen to the radio during the 5am-9am and 6am-10am hours, while they are in rush hour traffic. Even though you most likely will have a shorter interview time on the morning shows, you will have many more listeners, which is best for your business.

- The second group of shows to pitch will be the afternoon, followed by late morning, early afternoon, evening and lastly, weekends. Work through the shows in this order. Don't even count overnight shows since most people are asleep when they air.

Now that you know how to organize and work through the database, it is time to begin making contact with the producers. You will find a wide variety of shows and it is important that you know what each one means before you call. Organization is very important throughout this process, and you will be just that much more organized if you already know what you are looking for.

-**Syndication.** A syndicated radio show is broadcast on two or more stations simultaneously. Syndicated shows are like hitting the radio interview jackpot because you will be heard by a much larger audience with one interview. Examples of syndicated radio shows include Sean Hannity, Jim Bohannon, Bob and Tom and many others. When you first start out, you may not be invited to interview on shows of this caliber, but there are hundreds of other syndicated shows that you can pitch your show idea to. You will receive the same benefit of reaching several audiences in different locations at one time, so don't hesitate to at least try to get a booking on a syndicated show.

-Shock jock shows. These shows can go to the very edge when it comes to the decency rules of the FCC. Often they are edgy and controversial, but many viewers find them to be fun. As discussed earlier, it is important that you read the entire description in the database, not just the format; especially, when it comes to talk shows. Depending on the topics, you may decide to eliminate talk stations from your list of stations to call. Shock jock shows are usually extreme and in some cases, outright vile. They do have lots of listeners, but maybe not the audience you are trying to attract.

-Talk radio. Talk stations do not play music; they just do as the name suggests...talk. The programming in this type of radio station formatting will vary. But what they do have in common is that they do program guest interviews and have a wide listening audience. There is such a huge variety in talk radio topics that you will most definitely be able to find a radio show that is compatible with your business. The database that I have compiled will be helpful for you to know who is likely to listen to the station in which you are interested. The database will contain demographics that will give you insight into the audience of the station you are trying to target. It contains a comprehensive breakdown of listeners sorted by gender, age and other factors. Again, you want to make sure that the target audience of any given talk radio show is compatible with your business interests.

-Music radio. Most people that are trying to promote their business through radio marketing assume that music radio is off limits. However, while most music radio stations do interview guests in the music industry, many will give brief interviews to guests whom they feel will capture the attention of the audience; even if the guest is not in the music industry. Music radio is focused primarily on entertainment, so even if you are given a shot at an interview, you must convince the producer that you are able to present your business in an upbeat, lighthearted and entertaining manner. I suggest that you do put them lower down on the list of stations to contact, keeping in mind that they are a long shot at best.

-Public affairs. Public affairs radio stations receive their funding from various sources including commercial and public financing and individual contributions. These public broadcasting stations are operated on a local or national level, depending on the country and the radio station itself. I suggest that you avoid programs in the "public affairs" category primarily because they are not broadcast live but most every interview is taped and broadcast during the very early Sunday morning hours, when most people are asleep. However, if you want to get some practice at interviews as well as recommendation letters to add to your press kit, a public affairs radio interview may be a good idea.

-News radio. I can provide you with helpful guidance when it comes to news radio. The key to successful promotion on news radio is that you make sure to highlight how your business ties in with, or expands upon, events that are currently in the news. It is a mistake to approach a news radio producer about an interview based strictly on promoting your business. For instance, staying fit and healthy for a longer life is big news today. You would show the news station producer how your nursing coach business directly relates to the latest health stories in the news, perhaps citing examples of how your clients have improved upon their health through your coaching. Remember the media release document in The Nurse Expert Vol 1? This is your ticket. To be even more convincing, tie in a local angle about your business so that listeners in the area become interested. You will get the promotion you need because the host will most likely give the name and location of your business at the end of the interview.

Caller Based Shows

All over the country, there are radio shows that are caller driven. These shows don't book studio guests; instead the callers become the guests. They differ from regular talk radio shows because they are based entirely on the interaction between the host and the phone "guests" that call into the open phone lines. The host will invite callers, usually by sparking a debate or other comments on current news. You can use these shows to your advantage. First, you can make it clear that you have a lot to say about the subject, explaining that you are an expert in your field. You can then plug your business (although not blatantly) by mentioning that this is how you come to know so much about the subject. If done effectively, this puts you in the position of being not just another opinionated caller, but an impromptu "guest" that will most likely be invited back as an official, scheduled guest.

Take advantage of this free marketing option by listening in on live shows on the Internet from around the world. Listen carefully for opportunities to speak about your topic. Be prepared to call when the host opens the phone lines. This is a way to get practice speaking and get a nice plug for your business at the same time. It is very easy to find radio shows on the Internet that are streamed and broadcast on the station's website.

Targeting the correct shows to promote your nursing coach business takes some planning, but it can be accomplished. Remember to take the time to organize the potential stations into categories and best choices before you start calling. It is a waste of time to make contact with producers whose shows are not appropriate to your business. An excellent database such as mine will help you with this crucial step. It will provide you with great information about demographics, station locations and their target audiences, making your choice easier. Knowing about the different radio station categories ahead of time is also helpful. Whatever your nursing coach specialty, it is important to be fully prepared before contacting potential radio stations. I am an expert in health care promotion and pubic relations (www.PRHealthCareCommunications.com) and in helping many new businesses to set up websites that include media pages (www. MedicalMarketingSEO.com)

Must Know Tips on Contacting Radio Shows and Booking the Interview

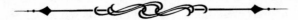

So far, we've learned about the advantages of utilizing radio marketing, several ways to promote yourself as an expert and how these interviews can catapult your business to the greatest heights possible. You know how to look for the appropriate shows and to have essential tools ready such as a fantastic press kit and an accurate and current database. I will now provide you with details on how to take that next step. In this chapter, you will learn what you can expect before, during and after the interview process. There are several things you must do before even making an attempt to contact a radio station, starting with becoming familiar with the show itself.

Tune in to the Radio Show in Advance

You will greatly increase your chances of securing an interview if you are familiar with the station and, in particular, the show on which you are trying to get an interview. In times past, this task was somewhat difficult since it was only possible to listen to radio shows broadcast in the area in which you lived. Thanks to the Internet, you can hear practically every station in the country in live time. All stations have websites that will let you log in to hear the programming right from your computer. The list of websites for major stations around the country is included in my extensive database. Use this tool to log on and get a feel for the shows in which you are interested. View this step as homework; the time spent listening will definitely pay off when you are ready to contact the show producers.

Your knowledge of the show's format, guest interaction and current events will let producers know that you have an interest in their station. Another convenient way to listen the shows is by downloading them, since most stations podcast their shows as well. This preparation in advance will avoid you showing up without preparation and insight into what goes on at the station, which can be a disaster for your interview and the way your business is presented.

Pre-written Pitch Script

For the same reasons you will not show up without knowing about the radio station, don't even think of calling the radio station without having a well written pitch script. Even the most experienced person needs to make sure their pitch script is down pat before picking up that phone. Keeping in mind that this may be your one and only shot at impressing the producer, do everything you can to make sure your pitch script is as perfect as possible. Write it as many times as you need to, then write it again to make it even better. Try creative editing so that it won't be too long, but be sure to leave in the major points.

Once you have the well-organized, professional and informative script in writing, you must rehearse it aloud. Practice saying the script until it comes out smoothly; many times what looks good on paper tends to sound choppy when verbalized. Continue to rehearse the pitch aloud and make changes as necessary. Then call a few friends and try the pitch out on them in order to get feedback. Once your pitch is perfected, you may want to try it out on a couple of the much smaller radio station until you are comfortable calling the larger station producers. The reaction you receive will give you an idea of whether your pitch is on the right track. For instance, if you keep getting interrupted by producers before you finish your pitch, it is probably too long. You can use this information as you continue to tweak the pitch to just the right timing.

Remember What You are Pitching

In my experience working with new private nursing coaches, I find one area where they consistently miss the mark. Many new business owners have a tendency to pitch their business to radio show producers. As discussed earlier, it is vital that you <u>pitch a show idea,</u> since the whole point of them interviewing you is to create an informative and entertaining show. During the course of the interview, you will undoubtedly be able to speak about your business and share your contact information, which is how your business is promoted. I am mentioning this at this point so that you will pause and think about it before you begin making calls. Remember, you are not trying to give the impression that you are interested in paid advertising, which is the impression you will give if you insist on promoting your business during the interview. I will be glad to give you individual help with developing a pitch that focuses on a show idea that will lead you to offers for interviews.

Keep Track of Your Calls

Whatever you do, make sure you keep an organized record of the calls you make. You can keep a call log right in the database that you will be using to make the calls from. Have the database in front of you as you make the calls. The log must be a very detailed, record of each and every call you make. Note the show that you called, the exact date, including month day *and* year, along with whom you talked to. Summarize what was said during the conversation, recording whether they asked for more information and, if so, when you sent the press kit or email they requested.

Keeping an accurate and detailed call log is one of the most important tasks you can perform in this process. In fact, without this log you will not be able to market your business on the radio effectively. You can very easily lose track of the people that you talked to and worse, forget to send out a press kit or other information that was requested. There are several ways to keep track of your calls. Some people use Microsoft Excel or another spreadsheet program. ACT and Access are other contact management programs that organize call logs. If you are not proficient at either making calls or keeping track of them, you may want to contract this work to someone else. Both of these services are offered by my company. If you do decide to have someone else make your pitch, there are several things you need to know.

Help with Pitching

There can be many reasons why it is best for you to have someone else pitch your business to radio station producers. Perhaps your schedule is far too busy; after all, the process does take a huge amount of time. Or, you may be shy about cold calling radio stations. Whatever the reason, you should realize that you are placing your business in the person's hands. It is the person (or company) that will make the first impression with the producer, so choose carefully.

Whoever will be doing your pitch for you must know your business almost as much as you do. They must believe in your business and have boundless energy and patience. As you can imagine, the person must be very personable and articulate on the telephone. Do not choose someone who has a tendency to be thin skinned, as they will most likely have a bad reaction to the many rejections they will face during the process. And most important, they must be extremely organized in order to keep an accurate call log. Ideally, you would make your own calls. However, if you choose to delegate this to someone else consider the following candidates:

- A spouse who meets the above requirements

- College interns

- Stay at home moms or dads (while children are at school and pets are put away)

- Contract employees from employment agencies

- Us! www.PRHealthCareCommunications.com

In addition to knowing all there is to know about your business, you should have the caller read this book in order to absorb all of the important information it contains. This will make them much more effective when they actually begin to make calls on your behalf. Another tip is to have them spend a day or two at your practice so they can experience what it is you do and how your practice is run. Just as if you were making the calls yourself, have the person practice the pitch and start calling the smallest stations first. Naturally, the pitch will be tweaked to indicate that they are calling the producer about a show idea on behalf of you. They will list your credentials and the show idea.

This tip is extremely important if you plan to use someone else to pitch on your behalf. Make sure you have a website that includes a media clip of you. This is because, without exception, the producer will want to know what *you* look and sound like; which they won't know from the person who is making the calls for you. When the person who is pitching for you calls the producer, they can advise them that a video clip of you is available on the website media page and invite them to take a look.

Before the person makes the calls, give them your exact times of availability. Give them the authority to make appointments and book interviews during available time slots on your calendar. This avoids the delays that would occur if they have to tell the producer they must check with you and get back. You want to make sure that you can get that interview on the spot. Train your pitcher to keep detailed information about each call, including what the producer said during the conversation. A little extra incentive such as a bonus may mean your pitcher will work even harder to get you booked.

The Best Pitches

Your pitch, as you well know, is the key that will open the door to your radio interview. As you have learned, you need the pitch to be perfect. Whether you deliver the pitch to the producers or have someone else do it, a perfect pitch must have essential characteristics. First, it must be short and concise. Pitches must also be relevant to a topic that the station believes will entertain or inform the audience. They should also be timely.

-**A shorter pitch is better.** The best pitches go directly to the point of the show. You (or your representative) should be able to get the producer's attention for a show idea immediately following the introduction and credentials. As a nursing coach, you (or your representative) need to be ready to throw that pitch without using up a lot of the producer's time. Let's try a practice run at a short pitch. In this example, you are a successful smoking cessation and RN Health Coach. You are listed on www.RNHealthCoach.com and have helped hundreds of people to lead healthier lifestyles by using the principles of L.I.T.E. Therapeutics, Inc.

You have a great website and a professional press or media kit. All of your ducks are in a row and you're ready to make your pitch. Assume the producer's name is John, and you've had the good fortune to get him on the phone. In this scenario, a short, effective pitch would go something like this:

> *Good Morning John. Thanks for taking my call. I have a quick idea for a show for you. Do you have just 30 seconds? [If yes, proceed. If no, simply ask a better time to call him back]. My name is --- [or I represent---]. I am an RN Health Coach who has helped over 500 twenty-year smokers permanently quit smoking. I am an expert in using my medical background as well as health education and encouragement to help long term smokers break free from smoking. Since the American Lung Association has designated this month as "Smoking Cessation Month", I would be great at providing strategies and inspiration to stop smoking for your listeners. I have an idea for a great segment called, "Is your smoking destroying your relationships? Learn 4 ways to stop this problem now!" If you are interested, I would be glad to send you a press kit along with my website address.*

Always make sure you ask if they have the time, even just 30 seconds. It shows that you respect their time and makes a very good impression. In addition, it saves you from irritating the producer or getting the phone hung up in your face. Because the truth is, the producer is so busy with all of the responsibilities that come with their job that it is possible they may not have even 30 seconds to spare. The key is not to make the pitch too long. Do not shorten the pitch by speaking quickly; just plan the pitch to say what you need to in as few words as possible.

-The show you pitch must be topical. Producers are hungry for shows that tie in with current events. How do you find show ideas that a producer will view as relevant? All it takes is keeping your eyes and ears open to current events. For instance, immediately following the holiday season is a good time to pitch your show idea for weight loss if you are a weight loss RN coach. You can include in your pitch that you will give the listeners tips on how losing weight can not only help them to live longer and look younger, but can also help with those post holiday blues many people tend to have.

Other topical show ideas can be found in the news, which is why you should make it a habit to stay on top of local and national news. The producers and hosts of radio shows continually seek to gauge the emotional status of their public. You can hear examples of this when the radio host will read news headlines and then solicit callers to weigh in on how they feel about the topic. It is a good idea to subscribe to news alerts through Google or other sources. Other topical show ideas can include contests, celebrities, politicians or other public figures. With a little imagination, you will see it is relatively easy to find ways to tie these subjects in with your nursing coach practice. I have had success helping RN wellness coaches to book radio interviews based upon local happenings such as job layoffs, violence in school and other issues that can affect overall health and wellness.

Timing is Everything: The Best Time to Call

The whole process of securing a radio interview should be carefully planned and fully organized. As you get closer to your goal, you want to ensure that you don't make missteps that could cost you the very marketing and promotion that you are seeking. Your initial call, as you've read thus far, can make or break your success. Therefore, in addition to being fully prepared with your pitch, you have to make sure you know the right times and circumstances to make your calls. While we've covered phone calls to radio station producers, there are instances when you will need to contact the host or even the Program Director. I will explain each of these people and the best times that you should call.

Producers

The role of the radio station producer is to book guests. As you can imagine, the producer is in constant motion prepping for the show, booking guests and other related tasks. It is true that it is the producer that you will usually call to pitch your show idea. However, let me give you some tips on the most effective ways to reach the producer.

- No calls before the show. Do not bug the producer just prior to a broadcast. I recommend that you do your homework and call within two hours after the show's end, which is usually how long producers stay at the studio. If you absolutely must call before a show, call no less than an hour before the show begins. You can find the exact show times in my comprehensive database.

- If you are not sure when the producer will be in, call in advance and ask what time they usually arrive. Every producer's schedule is different; many wear several hats, which may include news or program director.

- For weekend radio shows, start calling during the week. You will find out whether they actually come in during the week (most do) or if they are more accessible by email. This will give you the information you need to follow up.

Program Director

The Program Director is responsible for overseeing all show programming and making the final decision regarding the content and broadcast scheduling. The Program Director supervises the producer. On rare occasions, the Program Director can be called in order for you to get their take on which shows might be of interest to the producer. Some business owners, authors and others have found success using this strategy. I also have included the names of the Program Directors of the radio stations in my database. If you decide to call the Program Director, let he or she know that you have ideas for the show but are unsure which one their station would think is appropriate. Ask if they have any input on how you can pitch the idea to the producer. An added bonus to this strategy is that you can truthfully say to the producer that you have spoken with their Program Director (who is their boss) and received their feedback that your idea is a perfect match for their show. Then pitch your show as you learned earlier in this book.

Host

The rule of thumb for calling radio show host directly is that you don't, unless they know you personally. The host can be your first contact if the station is very small and the host is also the producer of the show, which is rare. As you move forward in your marketing, you may be invited to interview with a host that you've broadcast with before, which may be a situation where you can call the host directly. Even so, it can be extremely difficult to reach a host directly, not only because they are super busy, but because they are buffered with secretaries and operators who are trained to protect them from all but the most necessary calls. Another thing you should think about before you decide to call the host directly is the affect your actions will have on the producer. Going over the producer's head, so to speak, is a sure way to irritate them to the point of making sure you do not get a shot at an interview.

Phone Etiquette

As a nurse professional, you are well aware of how to behave in a professional manner. I am including this information since, in the excitement of the moment, you or your representative become unsure how to handle the phone call to the radio station. Even though you may be confident with your pitch, there is no chance you will dial the station and the producer will answer the phone. More likely, you will speak to an operator, secretary or even a voice mail machine. Depending on how you handle the conversation with the operator, you could make it harder on yourself than it need be to speak with the producer. I will teach you how to get from the station operator all the way to the producer.

Operator Do's and Don'ts

- Do remember that the operator is paid to do the job of screening and directing calls. A good operator will be as thorough as possible before directing you to the producer's office.

- Don't be rude or impatient with the operator. It won't get you anywhere, and besides, it is their job as the first line of defense to be inquisitive and protective of their employers.

- Do try to get the name of an operator that you have come in contact with, making a note in the database. Remaining friendly with an operator just might give you an edge when it comes to reaching the producer.

- Don't forget that if you are booked for an interview, the same operator will most likely field inquiry calls about your business. If you are respectful and friendly, they will most likely treat your potential client calls likewise.

- Do ask for the producer by both the first and last name when you reach the operator.

- If you happen to know a nickname that the producer goes by, using that name will impress the operator that you have spoken with the producer before.

Dealing with Voicemail

When you ask the operator for the producer and are transferred to the producer's line, you will almost certainly get the producer's voicemail, so be prepared. Leave your well-prepared but very short pitch on the voicemail. Make sure that you say your phone number and website clearly two times. Do not call again until two days have passed in order to give the producer a chance to return your call. Don't be discouraged if you don't get a call back, it happens all the time. However, there are methods you can utilize to increase your chances of getting a return call and they are not difficult at all. I will teach you the correct way to follow up on phone calls.

If you haven't received a call back after two days, call again. You will probably go through the same routine-operator then voicemail. This time, you should hang up and call back. Or, if there is an option to return to the operator, do so. When you speak again with the operator, politely ask if they would page the producer. The operator will ask who is calling and you should simply give your first and last name (with no further explanation) in a tone that suggests your call is expected, which usually results in a page to the producer. However, if the operator asks whether your call is expected by the producer, you should be truthful and so no. If asked what your call is regarding, you should say something simple like, to schedule an interview or regarding an idea for a show. Again, keep your tone authoritative and confident but very polite.

If after these attempts, the operator insists that you leave a message there or on voicemail, I suggest that you keep attempting to call and speak with the producer rather than leave repeated voicemail messages. But be persistent if the operator says the producer is on another phone call and request that you be placed on hold until the producer is free. If a week or more has passed without results, continue to call but leave only one message each week until the producer returns your call. This lets the producer see that you are excited about being a guest but are respectful enough not to bombard them with messages.

Email Blasts

Throughout this book, I have stressed the importance of contacting the producer in order to get radio interviews. But you may run into situations where alternative means of contacting the station become necessary. One such option is to send an email blast. An email blast is promoting your business by sending out simultaneous mass emails to promote yourself and your business. I have had success helping nurse coaches to promote themselves and eventually secure interviews with large radio stations by using email blasts, but only under specific controlled circumstances.

-**Trying out different show ideas.** In this situation, an email blast campaign can be compared to a fishing expedition. You send out the emails and see which ideas grab the most attention and results in responses. If you use an email blast to experiment with potential ideas, indicate in the subject line that the email is a show idea or pitch. Then hook the reader in with a catchy line, followed by the most compelling bullet points from your press kit. You can take it a step further by putting teaser lines with links to your website media page for further information. Do not send attachments in emails. Rather, direct the reader to your website. My medical marketing company can create a well-formatted, professional website that will include video and/or audio clips so that viewers can get a preview of your business.

-**Breaking news story.** Be prepared to send out an email blast the moment you are aware of a breaking news story that ties in with your business. I can't tell you how many people I have helped to benefit from using this strategy. This is among the reasons that I advised you to subscribe to a news service; jumping in while the topic is hot is a sure way to open the door to a radio interview. The best-case scenario is that you get a phone call or email in return and are invited to be a guest on a radio show. Most likely, however, you need to make a follow up call, preferably the same day. Ask the producer if they saw your email, it is possible that they have and are interested in interviewing you. If not, at least you've impressed the producer by showing you are eager to be on the show and willing to follow up with the station. At the very least, if they haven't seen your email, a call gives you a chance to make a good impression (and possibly give a quick pitch).

Sending Video Emails

Video emails are a high tech option to get your pitch heard by radio (or even television) producers. They can be quite effective if you go the extra mile to send each one personally, rather than all at once to several producers as in the email blast. I can help you to create video emails with techniques that have proven to be successful for many clients. However, if you are tech savvy, it is possible for you to create your own with a little effort. You will need a mini cam attached to your computer. Before you record, prepare and rehearse your pitch just as you did with the pitch you will be using for phone calls. It's as simple as recording the video message (keep it short) and sending to the email to the producer, which will contain a link to the video you've record it. A personalized video goes a long way in making a positive impact. Just as you would with an in-person interview, make sure you pay special attention to your appearance and how you speak. Also, be aware of the surroundings that will be visible in the video.

The Importance of Follow Up

No matter how many voicemails, messages or emails you have sent, you must be consistent and persistent in your follow up. You are responsible for getting the producer to speak with you, not the other way around. Do not take the easy way out and give up if you receive a no. If you adhere to all you've learned in this book, there will be countless times that you will be booked for interviews on the spot. But, as you can guess, there will be times when you will be met with resistance, delay or oven rejection. I cannot tell you how many times I have seen success with clients that simply refused to give up.

In my experience, most nursing coaches are booked after about six attempts at making contact with the producer. You must learn to exercise patience and get back on the horse, so to speak, when you have not received a return phone call. In fact, waiting for producers to call you can sometimes guarantee that you won't get booked. You must be relentless, but respectful, by taking your destiny into your hands and following up with the producer. Think of it this way. Follow up is the actual lifeblood of your business. If you cut off this crucial aspect, you will without a doubt watch your business dwindle because of its not being consistently promoted.

Remember, marketing and promotion is an ongoing process. The very first time you attempt to promote your business starts a cycle that does not end until you have booked that radio interview. Don't forget that there are so many others that are clamoring for the attention of radio show producers, many in your same industry. Commit to promoting yourself and your business each and every day. Tirelessly make initial phone pitches, email or video blasts, or other marketing efforts until you meet with success. Keep organized so that you can put this same continual effort into following up with radio stations that you have not heard from.

This part of the book puts you right at the door to ultimate success, so you must refuse to give up. For inspiration, keep in mind that you are receiving something very valuable for no cost. As you learned in the first chapter, free radio marketing can be a tool that can bring in more business than you can handle. Why risk missing out on your business taking off? Rather, dedicate yourself to following up on every phone call, email and other contact until it becomes second nature to you. If you need help with any aspect of your business, whether it is marketing, promotion and public relations or website development, visit either of my company websites at www.PRHealthCareCommunications.com and www. MedicalMarketingSEO.com. I am confident that I can provide the ongoing support you need to experience results well beyond your expectations.

When the Producer Shows Interest

If you have carefully followed the advice I have provided in this book, more than likely you will hear the words that you have been waiting hear from the producer; "we are interested". Do not question that you heard wrong; these words are evidence that your preparation, hard work and persistence have paid off. But again, be prepared for what will ultimately be the next statement, which is when the producer will ask, right then and there, for you to provide some more information about you, your experience and your business.

I will tell you that at this point the producer is conducting what is called a pre-interview; although they will never come right out and tell you this. The pre-interview is a test of sorts. The producer is weighing how well you interview, assessing your energy level and intelligence while making a firm decision about whether they will actually book you. I can teach you how to grasp this opportunity and make it work for you. You must first settle down and then realize the situation that you are facing. Have the mindset that you are in the actual interview live on the air. Put it in your head that you will not blow it-and you won't. Don't shy away from the weight of this moment in time. Instead, embrace it as the moment you have been waiting for. You are the best expert on your nurse coaching practice and this is actually the time for you to show off.

During the pre-interview is a good time to impress the producer with your versatility. Convey that you are an expert on several topics and how your flexibility can be useful in a wide range of show topics. As an example, if you are a nursing coach with a specialty in weight loss, don't limit your knowledge to topics such as diet and exercise. Show the producer that your vast range of experiences makes you an expert on total wellness, including the emotional issues that overweight people must deal with. This automatically puts you in line for interviews that deal with weight, emotional health as well as overall physical health, upping the odds that you will be chosen for this and subsequent interviews. Having said this, I must make it clear to you to stay on focus as much as possible with the topic of your initial pitch. Introduce your versatility without going so far out in left field that the producer is left confused.

Presenting yourself as a composed, intelligent and well-rounded expert reaps tons of positive consequences for you. I have seen many instances in which producers call upon nursing coaches for advice regarding their own health issues. So, whether you realize it or not, you are speaking with a potential client, who could recommend many more clients, during the pre-interview. This is another way that radio marketing provides you with free advertising to increase your business.

Producer Responses: "No" and "Later" and "Another Show"

Once the producer hears you pitch, either from you directly or on voicemail, most likely you will get some kind of response. We just covered the pre-interview and how to proceed if the producer shows interest. The producer will ask you for more information about you and your business, so be prepared with excellent press kits, a winning website and current contact information. For those occasions when you do not get an immediate "yes", you need to have a set plan to follow. Now I will teach you how to handle the other responses that you will encounter, which are "not interested", "perhaps later" and "another radio show".

How to Respond to a "No"

In an ideal world, you will be offered the chance for a radio interview each and every time you deliver a pitch to the producer. But, as you know, this is unrealistic and you will get the occasional "no, thank you". When a producer listens to your pitch and clearly lets you know there is no interest, do not attempt to bargain or convince at that moment. You should most certainly give them their space; let it go for a time while you concentrate your efforts on other potential opportunities.

But let me give you a couple of pieces of sound advice here. Although it may be helpful to reflect on how the pitch went in case you can sense ways it can be improved, do not obsess over it or lose your confidence. Do not take the rejection personally, even though you may feel slighted. Producers get literally thousands of pitches in any given month and it is their job to make what they feel is the best decision at the moment. The second piece of advice I can give you is to never assume that the no is a permanent answer. It could very well be that the producer needs time to think it over and does not want to risk that you will pester them if they say "maybe". Instead, think of it as a "no" answer that can very well be a "later" deferred, which I will go into detail about later.

If you have been given a negative response, learn from my experience about producers. Radio stations experience high producer turnover. Therefore, put your conversation in the log you are keeping, but by all means check back in six months to see if the station has changed producers. If so, this is an opportunity to start over with a new pitch, possibly tweaking your old one based on the comments of the producer who rejected your idea. The same principle can apply if the show hires a new host later; you can always try to pitch your idea to the same producer with a spin on it that you believe the new host will be more receptive to your topic.

But what if the producer, host and program director remain the same after six months? Should you give up on the station and delete them from your database? No, find the courage to contact the producer after six months. Come up with a slightly different angle to your pitch that might garner interest. You can also make a fresh approach by tweaking your pitch to include a hot topic that is in the current news. Or you just might happen to call when the station is looking for exactly the show you are pitching. At the very least, you will be politely but consistently keeping your name and show idea in their memory in case they want to use your show idea at a later date.

"Maybe Later"

You will also encounter producers that respond to your pitch with "perhaps we could interview you at a later time". As tempting as it may be, do not let your mind view this as a rejection, because it simply is not. What you need to do is shake off all insecurity and doubt and prepare for "later". Maintain your composure, do not reveal even a hint of disappointment or anger in your tone. Do not burn your bridge with this producer by giving off an air of dismissal. Politely ask the producer for what they believe is a good time frame to check back. Thank them for their time and then make detailed notes about the conversation in your database or however you are keeping track of your calls. Be sure to follow up as suggested by the producer. In the meantime, make any changes or additions to your pitch that will give you a definite answer the next time you call.

If the Producer Recommends Another Show

The producer might listen to your pitch and tell you that, although they are not interested, another station, show or producer might be willing to book an interview. Do not take this suggestion as a way to get you off the phone. Instead, listen carefully to the suggestion and get as much information about the colleague as possible. Trust me; if the producer recommends another producer, odds are they are familiar with that person as well as what that station may be looking for. In the event you are given a definite "no", take this tip even further by taking the initiative to ask the producer if the station has a sister station or whether they have a referral. You will be surprised how eager some producers are to do this, if only because they feel badly about turning you down.

Answering Questions about Other Local Interviews

Sometimes a producer will ask several questions before making a decision whether to book you. Often, the questions are as simple as whether you have a press kit, website or other information. But there are times when the producer will want to know if you have been interviewed by other stations in the area. Whether you have or have not had any interview experience or recently interviewed in the same area, don't start to panic. There are ways I can teach you to answer whatever questions you are asked.

If you have done interviews in the local area, answer the question somewhat evasively. Answer the question with statements such as "not in the recent past" or "yes, a while ago". If the producer presses you for a more specific time frame, don't feel as if they are picking on you personally. It is the job of the producer to keep their station "fresh" by being the first to interview guests. This is when you need to tread carefully, because some producers will automatically turn you down if you have been recently interviewed by one or more competing stations. Try to not give definite answers and never simply volunteer that you have made the rounds in the area just recently. However, do not outright lie because you will run the risk that the station will discover your deceit and you will definitely lose your credibility.

At this point, I would also like to caution you about sending your press kits. Take the time to consider each mailing on an individual basis; don't just send the press kit out without any thought because it has been requested. For the same reasons as I mentioned above, you will want to go through the press kit and take out any recommendation letters composed by radio producers in the same city.

Additional Tools for Booking an Interview

My commitment to you is to provide you with as many tools as possible for your success in radio marketing. You will encounter so many different issues that it may seem impossible to keep up. But take heart, I will utilize all of my expertise and experience in marketing to provide you with as much information as possible to meet and conquer each challenge. I will use this section of the book to cover a few miscellaneous issues that may arise while you are at the cusp of getting booked for that interview. This section will cover the following:

-Language Accents. It is important for me to address this issue for those of you who are concerned that your accent will cause problems on your radio interviews.

-Questions you should avoid. Of course, you need to make inquires before you decide to accept an interview invitation. But there are areas that you should avoid questioning until the timing is right.

-Moving through the station list. Never assume that you should simply go down the list in order to make your pitch calls. There's a definite method you should follow to save time and produce the best results.

-Language Accents. Since we live in a country filled with diversity, many of us speak with the accent of our native language. If you are wondering whether you will be able to get radio interviews because of your accent, let my company help you. I am fortunate to have clients from diverse backgrounds, ethnicities and nationalities. Believe it or not, it may be possible that your accent can work to your benefit, rather than hinder, your success.

The primary issue that the producer is concerned with is whether the station's listeners understand what the guest is saying. As far as that goes, it is equally important that the producer and the host can communicate clearly with the guest as well. As long as this requirement is met, then the issue of your accent is not a problem. But if you have an accent that makes it difficult for people to understand, we can start working with you to help.

One option to help with your accent can be to hire a speech coach that can work with you to help you speak English clearly. Language programs are also available that will teach you how to use English more effectively. The good news is that the ultimate goal is not for you to "lose" your accent. Everyone has an accent of some sort. Nevertheless, as charming as an accent can be, you have to be clearly understood. In many cases, your accent can be beneficial. For instance, if you are providing health information about eating or smoking habits in your native country, listeners will most likely find you more credible if you have an accent from the country about which you are speaking.

-Questions you should avoid. The biggest mistake you can make when you give your pitch is to ask the producer the size of their station. Do not ask the station's market ranking, wattage or number of listeners. First, this information will be provided to you in my extensive database, so you will not need to ask. In addition, grilling a producer about the station is not a good idea, as they may get the impression that you believe you may be too big for their station. One way you can gauge the size or popularity of a station is if the producer in a smaller town insists on providing you with the station stats. You will soon learn that stations that are well established and of a good size do not advertise their stats. If you run across a station, perhaps through a recommendation that is not in my database, you can always call the station and pose as an advertiser to get statistics about the station. But under no circumstances should you ask these questions during the pitch or pre-interview stages of the process.

-**Moving through the station list.** If you recall, we talked about how to make your pitch calls starting with morning show producers. Once you have thoroughly worked all of the morning shows on the list, it is time to start at the beginning of the list and call producers of afternoon shows. You will then repeat the process for midday and then weekend shows. Although this may seem repetitive, it is not because nothing says you cannot do interviews in different time slots with the same station. But - and this is important - do not volunteer the fact that you were interviewed on the morning show. Most producers do not want to create conflict with producers of shows airing at other times of the day.

Types of Interviews

Without a doubt, using the information I have provided, you will be invited to be a guest on a radio show. I will teach you some of the things you need to know so you will be clear just what you are getting into. In this section, I will cover the difference between taped and lives shows. In addition, I will provide an overview of what studio and over the phone interviews entail.

Taped and Live Interviews

Radio interviews are almost exclusively broadcast live. In most locations, the only stations that air taped interviews are music stations. If a music station producer offers you an interview, do your best to convince them that you are well prepared, exciting and professional enough to give an excellent interview. Music station producers prefer taped interviews because they are concerned that a guest will use foul language, freeze up during the interview, or say something offensive. I recommend that you do live interviews, even if the producer tries to convince you to tape an interview. In my experience, these are a couple of the primary reasons to choose live interviews over taped:

- Bearing in mind that you need as many people to hear you as possible, a drawback to taping an interview is that you have no say in when it will be broadcast. The worse case scenario is that it won't air at all, and even if it does, you risk it airing during a time when no one is listening. Here's a helpful tip: If you gave what you believe was a really good interview and it didn't result in any inquiries, it could be possible that it did not air at all, in spite of what the producer may tell you. Or, even worse, it aired without providing your contact information.

- A taped interview does not allow the variety that comes from taking listener calls. Without this feedback, you are unsure whether your message is being received by the listeners. You can sway a producer to allow a live interview by explaining that without taking listener calls they are robbing their listeners of an interactive experience with the station.

Even though you have a strong preference to do live interviews, you still may run across a producer that won't budge. If the producer insists on a taped interview, make sure you are not impolite or confrontational. If a taped interview is inevitable, politely let the producer know that you want your interview broadcast during rush hour or other peak driving hours. Nicely request that they leave in all of your contact information if cuts have to be made. Know when to give in to the producer before they change their mind about interviewing you. In many cases, the decision may not be the producers. Some stations have a strict policy to air only taped interviews, which is out of the producer's control. But whatever you do, don't agree to a taped interview without putting up at least some resistance.

Studio and Telephone Interviews

When you get booked for an interview, the producer will probably ask whether you can come to the studio to do the interview or only have phone availability. If given a choice, I would advise that you pick studio interviews, if the drive is not too far, for many reasons. First, you will get to meet the producers and hosts in person, which will come in handy for future networking and also offer you the chance to get photos to add to your press kit. Studio interviews also offer more airtime than taped interviews. I find that my clients gain an edge when they are open to doing studio interviews, since the majority of radio interviews are done over the phone. Even in top radio stations, the sound quality can be affected when interviews are done over the phone, which could reflect on your business.

An additional advantage of studio interviews is that you will be immediately provided with a recording of the interview, which is a reason to keep a blank CD or jump drive with you. In addition, traveling to the studio in person can also provide you with other interview opportunities with sister stations that occupy the same building, which is a definite bonus and can justify the drive.

When the Radio Station Contacts You

You will eventually begin to get calls from radio stations wishing to interview you. These calls are usually from referrals from other stations, or the producers have heard you and are ready to book you right away. After speaking with a producer who has called you, send a follow up email with a link to your website's media page. Sometimes a producer will contact you by email. If the producer has already made up their mind to book you, you may not get a phone call at all. In these instances, you don't need to send a press kit unless they ask for it before they book you. There are several types of stations that will most likely initiate contact with you.

-**Small or fledgling stations.** I will teach you how to handle an interview request from a radio station that is so small and amateurish it is not worth your time. In such cases, even though the station may be real dinky at present, it can grow into a big station in less than no time. Therefore, be very careful about how you treat the producer and don't turn down the interview if it is from a real radio station, no matter how small. The producer will be sure to remember you when the station grows into one of the largest in the area.

-**Nationally syndicated shows.** Nationally syndicated shows will very often call and entice you to do an interview based on how big their audience is, how many states they broadcast in and the number of stations that broadcast their show. If you recall, we learned that the transmitter signal of a station does not indicate how many people are really listening in. In actuality, if they cover a large area and have no listeners, they are no better than a tiny local station. Keep this in mind if you do an interview on one of these stations and do not get any inquiries about your business.

-Internet Radio Shows. There are two types of Internet radio shows, although neither are real broadcast shows. There are the legitimate Internet shows and the blatantly fraudulent shows. My expertise includes knowing how to spot the frauds, whose goal is to try to get your services for free. They can be easily recognized because they never give the call letters for their so-called radio station. I've seen them refer to themselves as radio networks that reach over a million listeners. But as I've taught you, it isn't how many people a station can reach, it is the number of people who are actually listening. When it comes to legitimate Internet radio shows, by all means it is a good idea to accept an interview if the topic of the show ties in with your business. If you are interested in doing the interview but somewhat skeptical, it won't hurt to ask the producer the number of verified listeners the station has and what those numbers are based upon. You may also request to talk to their past guests. These questions should give you an idea of whether the station is on the up and up, depending on their reaction.

-Satellite Radio. Satellite radio is really starting to take off and several big names have jumped on board. It still remains to be seen whether it will become as big as regular broadcast radio. But the point you are concerned with is which medium has the largest audience. I suggest that if a satellite radio station contacts you for an interview, that you do the interview. But since satellite radio is still in the growing stage, be realistic with your expectations about the results the interview will provide.

-Brokered Radio Shows. I am giving you fair warning that if a show asks that you pay to be interviewed on their show, it is most likely either not a real radio station or a shady operation. Think about this. If they are charging you to be on their show, they must not have any listeners. Otherwise, they would be selling advertising instead of charging guests money. The whole point of radio marketing is that it can promote your business at no cost to you. And there is definitely no shortage of free time slots for guests to be interviewed, over 10,000 each day by some estimates, and that's just in the United States. There are some people who sell airtime to guests while they are trying to start their own show, and many American radio stations sell airtime in 30 and 60-minute slots to real estate offices, attorneys, mortgage brokers and so forth. This type of "infomercial" style radio talk show is nothing new. However, for the purposes of promoting your new nursing coaching business, paying to be interviewed simply does not make sense and I recommend that you do not do it.

In the next chapter, we will cover valuable information about how to prepare for the grand prize - the actual interview! I will teach you all you need to know about the process including scheduling and how to prepare to present yourself and your business in the best light.

Preparing for the Actual Interview

A consistent theme throughout this book is to always be organized and prepared, no matter what step in the process you find yourself. And you must continue this when you reach your goal of booking interviews. Here I will go into detail on how to prepare for the interview using the following topics:

- **Keeping Track of Interviews**

- **Interview Scheduling**

- **Best Time Slots**

- **Advance Scheduling and Time Zones**

- **Confirming the Details of the Interview**

- **Addressing the Host**

- **Phone Interview Preparation**

- **Advance Preparation for an In-Studio Interview**

- **If the Interview is Rescheduled**

Keeping Track of Interviews

I advise clients to prepare an interview document to keep track of their interviews. This log will organize all of the information regarding each interview so that you can refer to it at glance as needed. The interview log can be created in a Word document, spreadsheet or any other format that is easy for you to use. Start filling out the information as it comes in, and complete the log after the interview. Whichever format you choose, I recommend your log contain spaces for you to note the following details:

- Call letters of the station

- Station and/or studio address

- Producer/Host names and other contact information such as emails

- The date and time of the interview

- The type of interview (live, taped, in studio or telephone)

- Take note of which cities the show will air and other station information such as the number of listeners, frequency, etc.

- Details about how you will be contacted on the day of the interview (if a phone interview)

- Any other reminders and notes such as if you agreed to give callers discounted rates, did you ask the producer to provide listeners with your contact information, etc.

- Take note whether this interview was a result of you contacting the station or if they called you

- Whether you sent a press kit or email

- If you followed up with a thank you letter

- Any other information that you feel you need

It is important that you are consistent with keeping an interview log. The log will not only help keep your current interviews on track and organized, but the information will be valuable to you going forward.

You can use the log to establish trends and patterns, and to look back to see your progress.

Interview Scheduling

You have followed your plan and everything is starting to come together. You are starting to get offers from radio stations for interviews, which was your ultimate goal. Allow me to give you some tips on scheduling your interviews that will prove to be in your best interests.

What are the best days of the week to interview? It is important that you have your schedule within view each time you make a call. After hearing your impressive pitch, many producers will ask then and there when you are available for an interview, so be ready. I advise my clients to avoid scheduling interviews on Fridays for a couple of reasons. If you recall, we discussed that most people listen to the radio as they travel to work. Commonly, they get to work and talk about what they have heard on the radio as they were driving in. If your interview takes place on a Friday, you limit the amount of days that you will be the topic of conversation (and you will) between co-workers. However, if you interview earlier in the week, people have the chance to share your show for several days without the risk of forgetting what they heard over the weekend. Many people who have done radio interviews have reported that the responses they receive correlate with the day of the week that their interview aired.

Best Time Slots

Now that you are learning to take your destiny into your own hands, apply these principles to even smaller details such as the time slot for your interview. When asked what time is good for you, state a preference rather than responding with whatever time is good for the producer. Naturally, you will be very excited and appreciative that you have been invited to be interviewed, but keep your wits about you and play it smart. If the producer has a morning show, choose the peak time between 7:30 and 8:30am. This is when most people will be listening. In fact, most people have arrived at work by 8:30 in their time zone and are no longer listening to the radio.

Always make sure you request this time slot in their local time, and tell the producer you're available during those hours on whichever day of the week they are available (avoiding Fridays as we discussed earlier). You should respond with a couple of options for the producer, and at that point ask which one of those works for them.

If you run into a producer who does not choose either option you've set forth, keep negotiating until you get a slot close to the one you prefer, even if it means you have to schedule a few days or even a couple of weeks later. The same principle applies to afternoon talk shows. The prime slot for afternoon interviews is 5:15 and 6:30pm. These are the times when people are driving home from work.

One more point about time slots. Most radio interviews end at the top or bottom of the hour (8:00 or 8:30). This is because network news feeds arrive during this time.

It is a good idea for you to book your interview to start a little past these times so that you can get a little more airtime. This especially applies to music stations.

Advance Scheduling and Time Zones

Do your best to schedule your interviews a week in advance so that you can have time to take care of your confirmation letter and any other information requested. It also gives you some time to get the word out in the local media about the upcoming interviews. But do not make the mistake of turning down an interview with a big radio station who wants to interview you sooner just to give yourself this lead time.

Even though you want to give yourself this advance time, don't schedule too far ahead. A good rule of thumb is about ten days in advance works best. I have seen instances where, unfortunately, the producer has completely forgotten about an interview scheduled far in to the future, despite secretaries and calendars. For this reason, sending a confirmation letter or email is a good idea as a reminder to the station as well as to you.

Be sure to keep up with the time zones for obvious reasons. And in cases where you are doing a very early morning interview, don't let the time zone difference show in your voice; make sure you are wide awake. If a producer seems hesitant to book you on an early show because they sense you may still be groggy, do your best to convince them that you have no problem because you wake up that early all the time.

Whatever you do, keep up with Daylight Savings time and the affects it has on states like Arizona and Phoenix, where the winter months are technically in Mountain Time and summer months Pacific Time.

Confirming the Details of the Interview

As you are confirming the details of the interview with the producer, there are certain "housekeeping" issues that should be performed. If possible, try to remember to get these details worked out to avoid having to contact the producer again prior to the interview. Again, this should be something that you do consistently with each interview so that you lessen the risk of forgetting something important.

-**Length of the interview.** Naturally, you will be curious to know how long the interview will last. Refrain from asking outright; usually the producer won't know anyway. The length will sometimes simply depend on how well you do with the interview. However, in order for you to avoid booking your interviews too close together, you do need a general idea of how long the interview will last. I suggest you ask about how much time the producer would like for you to block for them. In reality, you should expect that the interview will last anywhere from five minutes to half an hour. Talk shows last longer, but don't pass up a shorter interview. Make the best of the time to increase your chances of getting called again and promote your business.

-**Contact information.** Once the interview is scheduled, be sure to exchange all information needed to make contact. If you are doing a phone interview, give the phone number they should call for the interview, which may or may not be your regular number. In case they need to contact you about changes before the interview, make sure they have all of your contact information including cell phone and email. Confirm that you have all of their contact information, and include everything on the interview log that you have prepared. Most stations have a hotline number; make sure you have it in case there's a problem with any of the producer's other numbers. Ask for another emergency contact number if the hotline is a toll free number because some toll free numbers work in restricted areas.

-Promoting your interview. Don't hesitate to remind the producer that you would like for the station to promote your upcoming interview. Most stations will tease their listeners by building on a topic or guest before the show is broadcast in order to give a boost to their ratings.

-Giveaways and contests. Oftentimes, producers will ask if they can promote your business and increase their ratings by giving away free services to listeners. For instance, a call in show will have a contest that says, "25 percent off your first consultation to the 25th caller", or something along those lines. You should be accommodating to such requests rather than insult the station. In fact, view it as a complement that the producer is so impressed with your nursing coach practice and also as a chance to get the word out about your business. If you are concerned how to handle these requests, I will be glad to help you as I've helped many others in my promotion and marketing company.

Addressing the Host

Part of getting prepared for the interview is making sure you are following the station protocol. It is important that you ask the producer how the host should be addressed. More hosts than you know have nicknames that they prefer to be called during an interview. They do not want their real names used on the air because they may have established their brand based upon this nickname. But you also must know the full real name of the host so that you can send appropriate thank you notes after the show. Make sure you use the real name on the envelope of the thank you letter so that it is not mistaken for fan mail. Knowing the host's real name can also be useful in the event the host goes to another station.

You also want to get a little information about your host, if possible. While you are speaking with the producer, ask if the host has a personal interest in the topic. This can help you to make your interview more personable by connecting with the host. Alternatively, it will give you a heads up in case the host has had a bad experience with someone in your field; perhaps he wants you on the show for some type of debate. Above all, you want to be on friendly yet respectful terms with the host to have a good productive interview.

Phone Interview Preparation

Being fully prepared for a phone interview has different aspects than preparation for an in-studio interview. Don't be fooled into thinking that all you need to do is make sure you hear the phone ring. Rather, there are steps you need to take to ensure that your telephone interview goes smoothly and professionally. The day before your phone interview, put in a friendly and respectful call to the station and speak with the operator. Introduce yourself and explain that you are scheduled to be on the show the next day. Confirm that they have received your information card to make sure your contact information is available for people who will call the station for more information after your interview. Let the operator know there will be lots of calls from listeners who will need your website information or other information about your business. Explain that you're trying to make it easier to field the phone calls. This one phone call can be very helpful when people call the operator to learn more about you.

The preparation that is needed will depend on the time slot of your interview. If the interview will be during your working hours, be sure to isolate yourself in your office and make sure you are not disturbed. Since you will most likely be nervous, especially if this is one of your first interviews, don't rely on your memory. Keep some notes right where you can see them so you have a point of reference, if needed. Have a glass of water, pen and paper handy as well.

Many times, you will have phone interviews from home, especially when you are doing an early morning show in an earlier time zone. Some of my more experienced clients do little preparation; they just sleep until the phone call from the station comes in. I do not suggest this for the beginner, however. You should make advance preparation, including the suggestions in the previous paragraph until you have your interviews down pat. But, keep in mind that each interview will be somewhat different and be ready to make adjustments during the interview as needed.

Not everyone has an easy time waking up in the mornings, so if you are a slow riser, be sure to set your alarm early enough to get out the cobwebs before the phone rings. Make sure your voice is clear and friendly; a lot of times you will go live on the air right after saying good morning to the producer. Before going live, the producer may chat with you very briefly, possibly asking how you would like to begin the interview. If you prepared properly, you have already sent a list of questions they should ask, so you are prepared for the interview. You will then have a short pause after the producer says hello, followed by a series of clicks and then a the producer will come back to you in a much louder or clearer voice, which is an indication that you are live on the air.

Practically every host will ask you questions that you have prepared in advance. The questions (which you've prepared) will be geared to focusing (but not selling) on your services and your nursing coach practice. But be forewarned, there are some hosts that will come at you from an entirely different angle. But since you are an expert in your field, prepared in advance, you will know your topic so well that you will avoid embarrassment in answering any question related to the subject of your nursing coach practice.

I tell my clients that the best thing to do is to commit to staying calm despite being nervous, since nervousness is natural. When you first begin, it may seem scary to know that millions of people are listening to you. This is one reason I have suggested that you start with smaller stations.

In either event, avoid thinking about anything except the conversation. Focus on the conversation the same way you would when talking with a friend. Even breathing helps to reduce nervousness, so remember to take slow breaths to combat the butterflies and you will be just fine.

Advance Preparation for an In-Studio Interview

The logistics for your in-studio interviews are different from phone interviews in many ways. Naturally, you will want your appearance to be appropriate, so plan what you are going to wear in advance. I suggest to my male clients that they not wear a suit and tie but a nice pear of slacks (or even really nice jeans) paired with a shirt or sweater. Women can dress comfortably in slacks or dresses (not formal) of their choice. Overdressing will make you very uncomfortable while driving and during the interview. But in order to be completely sure, I advise that you take your cues from the station itself. You can either ask directly or go on the station's website and see how the hosts are dressed and wear comparable clothes.

Pack some of your press kits and a blank CD or jump drive in advance, so you won't forget to bring them. It is also a good idea to bring another copy of your sample questions just in case the producer has misplaced the copy you sent. Bring along a camera to take pictures with the host or of yourself at the microphone to use with your press kit. Extra copies of your information cards should be with you in case they are needed.

You will be traveling on the road, so you first want to ensure that you leave early enough to reach the studio early. The weather, accidents, heavy traffic or any other situation can put you in danger of being late for that important interview. Before you leave, make sure you have a fully charged cell phone, road map and studio hotline numbers with you in case you are delayed or if you get lost. Confirm you have the proper instructions for parking and security before you reach the studio.

Your goal is to reach the actual studio a little early to give yourself time to get logged in with the receptionist and guard, go to the restroom if needed, and relax with a glass of water after you meet the host and producer. In some of the larger radio stations, security is very strict, so you may be delayed while you pass through security. You want to be in a relaxed frame of mind when the interview begins and taking a few minutes to go over any notes you may have will help to boost your confidence.

While it may be acceptable to bring an adult companion with you for support and to take pictures, make sure that they are not in the way. Never bring children or pets, unless they are pre-planned as part of the topic of your show.

If the Interview is Rescheduled

I want to prepare you in the event your interview is rescheduled or delayed by the station since you will most likely encounter this at some point. In this section, I will teach you how to respond to receiving news that your interview has been temporarily cancelled. Among the reasons a radio interview may be reschedule are:

- Major sports event
- Late breaking news
- Foul weather
- Famous celebrity scheduled at the last minute

It is imperative that if you are informed that your interview is rescheduled, for any reason, that you respond positively. Let the producer know that you understand and look forward to the interview later. There may even be an occasion when they may not get the chance to give you advance notice. A few of my clients have had the experience of being at the studio, waiting for their interview, and not been called. If this happens to you, wait until maybe 10 minutes past your interview time and politely inquire whether you still going to be on the show. The issue may be that the station is simply running behind in their program schedule. Or, there may have been a mistake in when you were scheduled and you were given an incorrect time. But it is possible that they have filled your time slot with another guest. Again, do not take offense, this is a common occurrence in show business. Believe me, if you respond with an angry, whining or complaining manner, the temporary delay will become permanent because you definitely will not be called back.

By all means, feel free to initiate the suggestion for rescheduling if it will make you late for another interview or important appointment. Sometimes, the station will be relieved; especially, if they have made a mistake in schedule. In this case, if they cannot reschedule you on the spot, accept that they will call you when the show is over to set up another time - if you have handled the situation correctly. Be proactive if you don't hear from them in a reasonable amount of time. It is perfectly acceptable to follow up on rescheduling. This persistence will pay off with a future booking. Don't panic if your interview is rescheduled or delayed. Use that time to prepare for the interview that will be the reward for keeping a cool head when the initial interview was delayed.

Now that you are prepared for your interview, I will teach you some secrets on how to make it the success you want it to be. You will learn how to get over your nervousness and be an entertaining guest. The next chapter will cover topics about how and when to speak, ways to control your emotions and how to deal with audience calls. Following the tools in the pages of this book will lead you to becoming a polished and successful radio show guest.

Secrets to Conducting a Great Interview

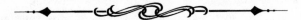

The moment you have worked so hard for has finally arrived. When you begin your first interview, you will feel a mixture of pride, excitement and nervous energy. Remember to remain confident that you have not reached this destination by accident. Now is the time for you to take charge and put your best face forward to promote your nursing coach practice as effectively as possible. In the excitement of the moment, you may find yourself wondering, what does the station want from me? What are their expectations of me during this interview? I can you tell that, without exception, you will be expected to be a passionate, energetic guest who is an expert on your subject matter. So long as you do not go through the interview with a depressing, insecure or arrogant demeanor, you will please both the station and the listening audience, which can only mean more success for your business.

Adapting Your Speech

As you continue to do interviews, you will be dealing with a variety of radio shows - some news shows, others may be music shows, humorous and lighthearted as well as serious topics. Beginning with that first pitch call, you want to make sure that you adapt your language to fit in with the feel of the station, particularly the way the host speaks. Earlier in this book, I pointed out the importance of listening to the station before you make the pitch call and this is one of the reasons why. It gives you insight into how the host speaks (formally or informally), and what type of audiences tune in to the show.

You must be comfortable with all types of people and situations. For instance, as a registered nurse you are familiar with lots of complicated medical terminology. If you are on a show that has an audience primarily made up of young listeners or other non-medical people, you must be careful that during the interview you do not speak "over them", using words that would be impossible for them to understand. Speaking in non-technical language about your business will win over audiences from a variety of backgrounds and education levels. Even other medical professionals will enjoy your interview more if you speak plainly. Learn to gauge whether you will be addressing a more sophisticated audience in order to adjust your speech accordingly. In other words, you must strike the correct balance between speaking on the audience's level without appearing condescending.

Have you ever watched a court trial on television and a so-called "expert witness" is called to testify? If the witness is a doctor, police officer or medical examiner, often their speech is so formal and hard to understand that they lose the attention of the jury, who are not usually members of these professions. Try to think of the same scenario when you are on the radio. Speak to the host, following his or her lead, but keep the audience that will be listening in mind. The odds are that the audience is not made up of your peers, but individuals who have an interest in their health or the health of their loved ones. Use common words and phrases even when you are not speaking about medical issues to keep the tone conversational. For example, using words like "saw", "started" and "went" flow more easily than using "observed", "commenced" and "proceeded", which sound much too formal for an everyday conversation.

Start of the Interview

Most interviews start with the host giving a brief introduction based on the bio in your press release. The host will then address you by saying "welcome", "thank you for coming" or something like that. You should make sure you give a brief but polite acknowledgement such as "thank you for inviting me" or something along those lines. As your interview experience grows, you can graciously add that you are a fan of the show (if you are) or some other gracious line. And with this begins the official start of your interview.

Some hosts start the first exchange by asking you how you began your career as a nursing coach. Or the host may ask what made you decide to open your practice. Do not hesitate in your answer. Use the next minute to toot your own horn. Talk about your credentials, experience and how you incorporate these into your practice. Give the audience a story of why you are so passionate about being a nursing coach. Relating stories of how it personally ties in with your life will provide a connection that both the host and audience will be drawn to. For instance, if your practice is focused on smoking cessation, you can convey your connection if you are a former smoker. Once you have established your background and what brought you to where you are today, you will continue the interview. Throughout the interview (with the questions you provided in advance), you will give the audience helpful information that they can use.

Some introductions, especially on shows where listeners call in, may begin a bit differently. As soon as the broadcast goes live the host may say something like, "we have (your name) on the phone and (your name) is here to tell you how to (lose weight, stop smoking, whatever is your specialty)". This lead in is intended to entice listeners to stay tuned in. You will not want to jump right into the information, but start off with saying something along the lines of how you will share how to (whatever the topic) but first you would like to share a little about who you are and your background. This is a means of controlling the interview, which I will teach you more about later in this chapter. At that point, the introduction will usually proceed as outlined in the previous paragraph.

Another introduction option is for you to write a script for the host to read just before you join him or her live on the air. If you prepare an introductory script, and the host agrees to use it, make sure the host plays up your expertise in your field. The host could say something like "The special guest, (your name) that we promised is here. (Your name) is a specialized nursing coach and owner of (your business). (Your name) will tell us how to (your specialty). Then the host will thank you for joining in and the interview will commence. This type of introduction gives you a chance to jump right into the essence and purpose of the interview.

If you decide to prepare an introductory script, make sure the script conveys the benefits of staying tuned in to hear the interview. The script should be composed with bullet points and include a separate document that clearly states that it is the introductory script of (your name) which is to be read by the host on the air just before the interview is read. You can either email the script to the producer or include it in the press kit.

Asserting Yourself in an Interview

Even though each interview is different and may have unexpected twists and turns, they have a somewhat common flow. Since this involves you and your business, you must ensure that it goes smoothly and that you convey all of the important points necessary to promote your business. You should never just sit back and let the host control the flow of the interview. Doing so will most certainly lead to you being disappointed about how it turns out. Instead, be proactive in dictating your destiny, especially since you have come so far in doing so.

Being passive and shy during an interview is a recipe for disaster. Do not wait for the host to lead you, although it is appropriate to let the host start off the interview as we just learned. Don't lose sight of the fact that the purpose of all of this is to advance your own business agenda. Deliver your information with passion; you will be surprised that a lot of hosts actually prefer you to do this. They will give you the reins (if you take them) and then just jump in with a question every now and then during the interview. I will teach you how to strike a balance between being assertive and coming off as rude. Once you have learned to do this, you will have tons of people who listened to the show contacting you.

In order to feel confidence with yourself during the interview, make sure that you have prepared a list of the important points you want to convey to the audience. Include the bullet points in the press release you prepared. Put the most important point at the very top of the list and work from there. Then, read and rehearse these points until you can communicate them in your sleep. Knowing what you want to say and how you want to deliver it is a surefire way to make your interview really count. You should never be passive and wait on your host to make the move. Don't lose sight of the purpose of all this, and so it is up to you to lead the host (and the audience) where you want them to go.

I can only give you the overall format of an interview as I have seen from my experience. Every interview will have small differences. There will definitely be mishaps and unexpected issues since interviews are not an exact science. And as you evolve in the radio marketing process, you will adjust how you handle your interviews. Eventually, you will walk away from your interviews confident that they went very well and served their purpose, so keep trying.

Tapping into the Emotions of the Audience

Even though I have been encouraging you to be passionate about your work in order to have a successful interview, I must explain how to keep your emotions under control. Emotions are very important, both yours and the emotions you trigger in the listening audience. If you use this power to strike an emotional chord with the audience carefully, you will have people calling you non-stop. Radio is show business, so you might as well learn how to use this to your advantage if you are going to use it to market your business.

There are several primary emotions that the listeners will respond to. They are greed, hate, anger and fear. Here I will discuss each one individually and how they can be used to get your desired results.

-Greed. Greed can also be described as want or desire. It is an extremely powerful motivator, whether people are trying to save money, earn extra money, or get something for free. Use this knowledge to reel in your listeners using greed as bait. For instance, you can offer free or reduced cost consulting or other services. You can also mention on the air that if they refer others to your practice they will receive (gift, free services or whatever). Trust me when I say that triggering the greed in people is an excellent way to increase your client base.

-Hate and Anger. These are among the strongest of human emotions. There are certain issues that most people strongly dislike, even to the point of hate and anger. Injustice, abuse of the sick and elderly and even authority are things that in some cases can automatically draw out a very strong reaction. Again, use this human emotion to the best advantage that you can. I must stress that this does not mean that you should make getting people angry the sole purpose of your interview. You especially do not want the listeners to be angry with you. What I am referring to here is tapping into the anger that most humans feel when they are treated unfairly. In your profession, you will come across many examples where you can use this in your interviews. For instance, if during your nursing career you have witnessed incidences of medical neglect or abuse, or even simple medical misinformation, either personally or from news stories, you may be able to tie this into why you decided to start your own nursing coach practice in order to give people affordable and accurate care possible.

-Fear. Of all emotions, fear is the one that motivates humans the most. But how can you tap into this emotion without scaring the radio audience? As it relates to your nursing profession, my answer is to first simply realize that people already have fears about their health. In fact, fear may be one of the main reasons they decided to tune in to the broadcast. This works in your favor because it is not you that has instilled the fear, but you can be the person who is an expert on how they can better manage their fear and their health. Because you will gain their respect just on the basis of being an expert nursing coach, all you have to do is use their fear and respect and offer them understanding and possible solutions to their situations.

Controlling Your Own Emotions During the Interview

As a radio show guest, you are somewhat at the mercy of the station and the host. In most interviews, the host will let you flow along and be in agreement with every word you say. But don't lose sight of the fact that you are in the show business arena and the goal for the host is to make sure the show is good at all costs. So you may come across a host whose agenda is to spark debate between the two of you or between you and the listeners. Some may deliberately disagree with a point you make in order to spice up the show. My advice to you is not to take it personally. Don't back down from your point, even if it means you find yourself in the middle of a debate. Once the interview is over, you will make up with the host in a professional manner and the two of you will probably have a good laugh together. You've seen this behavior in court cases when opposing attorneys go head to head in the heat of the trial and then go out for a drink together at the end of the day. It is the same with you and your host; don't let hostility build up to the boiling point. Remember that it is all part of entertaining the listeners and not a personal assault against your or your profession.

Interacting with the Radio Host

I have taught many of my clients how to take charge during the interview. Earlier in this chapter, I even mentioned that you might want to keep talking until the host interrupts you with a question. But I would like to clarify the parameters of how to interact with your host. Do not make the mistake of just going full force through your points and ignoring your host. Besides turning your interview into a commercial, you will most likely not be invited to interview in the future. Instead, interact with your host by doing a verbal dance while the two of you work your way to the meat of the interview (more on that later). Remember, your host will be doing the talking first during the introduction. Make the transition from the introduction to the interview flow smoothly, even if have to ask a question in order to draw them back into the interview once you get going. The key is to take control of the interview without ostracizing the host. As you gain experience, you will learn how to gauge the type of host you are dealing with. Some hosts are excellent at what they do, others not so good. You will run into hosts with huge egos who do their best to undermine you, while others are confident enough to let you take the lead in the show. Just be ready to adapt to both the host and the situation and remember that no matter what, you are a guest on the show.

As you go through the interview, remember to keep your conversation with the host and not the radio audience. In a radio interview the host will speak directly to the listeners; it is not your role to do so. The host has invited you to be on their show and as you recall, they will welcome you to the show in the introduction. Don't make the mistake of saying something like, "Hello listeners, I want to tell you about (whatever the topic). This type of behavior is an insult to the host. Think of it as being invited to a party and pulling all of the party guests to a party at your home, leaving the host home alone. Let me show you how to interact with the audience once the lines are open to listener calls, which is a different situation entirely.

How to Handle Calls from the Audience

If you are on a radio show in which the host opens the line for callers, you must be fully prepared in order to handle this situation. This will often happen on talk radio stations and can prove challenging if you are not prepared. This is because, unlike the scripted introduction or the preparation you've done to include important points, calls from listeners are totally unrehearsed. I encourage you to take this as not so much a disadvantage but as a chance to have a little challenging fun. The best piece of advice I can give you on this subject is to make sure you have your topic and material down pat at all times. Trust me; it will pay off in dividends when you start to field unexpected calls from listeners.

Most music station producers and hosts will ask in advance for your approval on taking listener calls. I suggest that if given an option, that you not do so until you are much more experienced in doing radio interviews. This is because you will inevitably get calls from irate or rude callers or someone who will take up precious time on a meaningless question. With experience, you will be able to handle these types of calls without being rattled. If you are given the option whether to take calls or not, politely let the producer know that you have a wealth of information to share with the audience and you would like to be able to share it during the limited that time you have for the interview. There will be times when taking live calls is unavoidable. I will show you how you can best handle this inevitability.

The first thing you should remember when taking live calls is to address the caller by their first name. You will most likely have help with this since the station's screener will display the first name and line on the host's screen. The host will usually say the first name and line number followed by "you are on the air with (your name), what is the question? Try to say hello to the caller before they begin speaking because it is the polite thing to do and will throw the caller off guard if they are calling to debate or argue. Unfortunately, the sole reason for a few callers will be to use you to vent their anger over something that has happened to them in the past, such as poor or inadequate medical care to them or a loved one.

If the caller has a reasonable question that you can answer, do so efficiently in as little time as possible. In the unlikely event you are asked something about which you have no knowledge, or have a problem answering, feel free to let the caller know that the question goes beyond your professional scope and that you are not an authority on that particular subject. Then follow this response by indicating that you are, however, knowledgeable about (related subject) and then proceed from there.

As unfair as it may seem, the wrong caller can actually break down your credibility. It is up to you to perform damage control and handle the call so that it turns around in your favor. Never play tit for tat with a caller; some will try to bait you to get into a heated argument. However, feel free to correct a caller in no uncertain terms when you feel it is necessary.

Watch your host for cues on how to handle certain callers; the host's attitude will pretty much show you whether the caller should be tolerated or not. I understand that this is all new to you. There will be occasions when it is best to just let the caller vent their emotions without you stopping them. Try to remember that you will become more proficient at listener calls as you gain more experience and practice.

The Core of the Interview

By this time, you have a good idea of how the interview will begin. We've covered the introduction and other parts of the interview, including audience participation. And while I have encouraged you to flow along with the interview format, I want you to never lose sight of why you are participating in the interview, and that is to use the show to promote your business. As such, you must be sure to cover certain points in order to garner interest in your business, despite other distractions or debates. These essential points of the interview, also known as the "meat", usually start just after you have done your introduction.

Again, no interview is the same, so with practice you will learn just when to begin this portion of your interview. If you recall, the points will be based on the bullet points in your press release. Ideally, these points will include your successes with your clients, how these were accomplished and how your audience can meet with the same success; among other core elements. As I've explained to you, practicing what you will say during the interview ahead of time will ensure that you don't miss important details. It will also help you to get your timing down pat, so you don't risk having to get cut off because you've run out of time.

I recommend to my clients to take, on average, one minute or a little more on each point. I refer to these as verbal bullet points. These are your one liners you learned about in *The Nurse Expert Vol. 1*. Radio stations call them sound bytes, or more literally, small pieces of information that are easy for the audience to absorb. Examples of these bullet points include:

- Statistics
- Humor
- Short stories
- Examples

You can use the exact points you want to make in one of these formats to make them more interesting and entertaining. For instance, you can begin by quoting statistics on the number of smokers just as you explain your smoking cessation program.

What is important is that you are educating the listeners while you are entertaining them. Combining these two elements will have much more impact that simply lecturing the audience.

Set your objective for the interview by picking two or three focused messages you want to stress. Listen for opportunities where you can reinforce your points via your one liners, focus points or sound bites.

Use these three steps to answer questions:

Step 1. Open answer with a simple statement, such as "That's right", "Absolutely", "no, no really", "Yes, it's true", "that's a common misconception"

Step 2. Give detail for support. Use bridging statement and transition into a short anecdote, professional or personal example, expert quote, statistic or fact. Explain what any facts may mean. Here are some effective bridging statements:

-"What's important to remember is…"

-"That reminds me…"

-"Even more importantly…"

-"You should also know…"

-"What I want to make sure you understand here is…"

Step 3. Identify a keyword given by the interviewer's original question. Link this keyword to a relevant and prepared message point. End with a benefit and or bridge to one of your key message points. Here are some effective statements that will lead you to your conclusion:

-"That is why we believe..."

-"The important point here is..."

-"and that is the best part about..."

-"What that means is..."

-"When we look at all those facts that I just laid out for you..."

-"We are going to keep doing exactly what has brought us our success..."

Keep your sentences short. Short sentences are stronger, powerful and more memorable. Aim for an average of 20 words or less for each sentence.

Message points

Before your interview prepare 3 message points you want to convey. Each message point should take about 10 seconds to say or be about 20 words in length. Be sure to include only 3 message points. Every question you answer will always bridge back to one or all of your message points. Your 3 message points will be repeated over and over so that your message is delivered. Of course you will not always say your message the same way every time. You will mix up the order, use different words, different examples.

Have a question you can't answer or simply don't want to answer? Use these steps:

Step 1. Address questioner by name.

Step 2. Use a bridge response. "The really important issue we should be talking about is.." "Clients would be better off if they asked about

..." "That's not the critical issue here. The critical issue is..." "That's like comparing apples and oranges. We can't be compared"

Step 3. Bride into one of your one liners, focus statements or sound bites.

How to Promote Your Business Discretely

Unless you promote your business, the whole interview is pointless, at least as far as you are concerned. But it would be disastrous if you turn the interview into a long boring commercial full of obvious plugs about your nursing coach practice. PR Health Care Communications, my marketing and promotion company, helps nurses like you learn to strike that perfect balance when they are being interviewed. There are two ways to get your practice out there in a discrete yet effective manner. They are plugging (or mentioning) your services and name repetition.

-**Plugging**. There's a skill to know how to get a plug in during the interview. I'm sure you already know it would be inappropriate to just openly solicit listeners with every other sentence you speak. You can plug your services by weaving references to your business and stories about successful clients throughout the core of the interview using the verbal bullet points. We touched on this in the last section, but I will go into a little more detail here. For instance, let's say the host asks you how you help clients who have been smoking for decades (assuming your coaching practice is smoking cessation). You could reply with an anecdote about an 80-year-old client that smoked for over 25 years and just celebrated his 5th year of quitting smoking (or a similar true story). Then you could follow up with "and this is how I helped him", and outline some of your services. In this manner, you are doing several things at once. First, you are giving smokers that are listening hope and inspiration. You are gaining credibility and educating the audience when you explain your services. And lastly, you are plugging the types of services you offer. Notice in this example how smoothly you can plug your services without shouting, "this is a commercial!" at the listening audience.

-**Repetition.** As human beings, one of the most effective ways we learn is by repetition. In the business world, branding is essential because potential customers repeatedly see the same identifier of a company and relate it to the business without even thinking about it. During the radio interview, you should mention your business name at least a couple of times, if possible. As with the plug, you want to integrate the name seamlessly into the conversation, unless the host asks you outright to tell the audience the name of your company.

Commercial and Other Breaks: How to Handle Interruptions

During a radio show interview, commercial breaks, music or other items will cut into the flow of the conversation. Don't let these interruptions throw you off your focus as they are inevitable. Although you may be somewhat new to radio interviews, trust that your host will know how to transition by taking these breaks during appropriate moments without leaving you in the middle of a sentence. Since you are fully prepared, there is no reason to get flustered and you will master the art of picking up after a break before long.

I discussed the important of small bytes using your bullet points earlier in the chapter, and this is one of the reasons why they are important. If you are in the middle of an important point you want to make and it is long and dragged out, you run the risk of the host having to cut you off to get in a commercial or other break. But this can also sometimes happen even when you are making a short point. Sometimes, the host will deliberately let you run close to the break time and then say something like, "Hold that thought. We will learn exactly how (such and such) when we return from the break, so stay tuned." Again, don't let this throw you off; the host is not being rude. This type of cliffhanger is known as a "teaser" and it is a way to keep listeners interested and tuned into the station.

Whether the break is a commercial, song or any other interruption, the station will let you hear what is broadcast to the audience so that you and the host know when it is time to resume the interview. Most often, the producer will keep track of how much time you have left and let you know in intervals how much time is left. Some guests use these breaks to take a restroom break or get a drink.

This is also a time when the host might have a little chat with you off the air. You can use this time to get the all important feedback from the host on how the show is going. The host may sometimes even share stories with you about their personal experiences that may relate to nursing. These breaks also help to build a connection between you and the host. Be friendly and outgoing with the host and be sure to compliment the station and their work. The break can also be a good time to ask if you can plug your business. If the show takes calls from listeners, the producer will most likely let you know about callers that are waiting to interact with you. Since the callers are screened before the get on the air, the producer will let you know the caller's question and allow you to choose whether to take certain calls. While this is not always the case, when you are offered this option you can believe, as the guests, your instruction will be followed.

How often does a station take a commercial or music break? Truthfully, this depends on how much money the station makes. The station may take a break every 10 minutes or half hour. Depending on the type of station, there may be interruptions caused by traffic updates, news or weather. When you interview on a talk radio show, the breaks are usually for one or more of these reasons. These breaks usually last under ten minutes. But on a music station, you, the guest, are actually referred to as "the break". These stations are on the air to play music, so your interview is actually the interruption in the programming.

Whatever the reason for the interruption, just stay relaxed and enjoy the break. Stay calm, regroup yourself so that you are ready to continue and complete your interview successfully. Clear your mind of any distractions that the interview may have caused. Bring your thoughts back to the reason you are there, which is to promote your business while keeping the audience entertained and informed.

The Conclusion of the Interview

How the interview closes is just as important as the introduction. These are the moments when everything you've done so far is summed up into a few minutes. How the interview is concluded is the last impression the listeners will have of you and your business. Most likely, it is most of what they will remember about the entire interview and will influence whether they contact you or not.

As the end of the interview draws closer, the host will say something to indicate that time is almost up. The host will address you and ask how people can find out more about you and your company. Just like during the introduction, this is your time to give it all you've got. You have learned throughout this book that preparation is everything. The same is true for your conclusion. You will want to have a well-rehearsed closing script committed to memory. Your conclusion is the time when you tell the listeners how they too, can receive the benefits of your fantastic nursing coach services or similar nursing service. You want to give them your contact information, including phone number and website address. In other words, it is the time in which you give a "shameless plug". You can also encourage them to reach you through the station, if you have been given permission to do so. There are several methods you can use to make your conclusion more effective, which include:

- Don't forget to speak clearly and slowly. This may take some advance practice. Start rehearsing the pace and clarity of your speech at home. Look in the mirror as you rehearse. Then close your eyes and get an idea of how you might sound to the listening audience, who will hear and not see you. Adjust as necessary until you feel you are easy to understand with a pleasant tone but in your natural speaking voice.

- Repeat your contact information twice. Assume that someone who is listening is trying to either write the information down or put it in his or her smart phone or other device. More commonly, listeners who are driving may be trying to commit the information to memory so that they can contact you when they have the time. Repeating it twice will also let you hear if you made a mistake when you gave out the information the first time.

- If you have an 800 number which includes a catchy vanity phrase (ex: 1 877 3-RN-Coach), say the word version first, then spell out each letter and then repeat it with numbers only ("that's 1 877 376 2622"). I suggest that you really try to entice people to come to your website, which you can do by offering certain advantages (more on this later).

- Save time by giving out the website address without saying the "WWW"; it is no longer necessary. Along the same lines, there is no need to say, "My toll free 800 number", as it is redundant since all 800 numbers are toll free.

- If you offer flat rates for certain services, you may mention how much these services cost. For instance, you may say that the cost for five weight loss coaching sessions are (name the price).

If you interview on a music station, you will probably only get the one chance to plug and that is as the interview is ending. Radio talk show interviews, which can last for one hour, usually provide the opportunity for at least two plugs, at the half hour and at the end. If you have developed a good rapport with your host, you can request that they set up a lead in for a plug just before the break. However, do not allow the interview to be mistaken for an infomercial, so deliver your plug in a discrete manner.

If for some reason the host forgets (or omits) to lead you into plugging your business services, assert yourself by mentioning your contact information anyway, even if it means cutting of the host from speaking. If your host starts to sign off without you getting in the plug, say something like "(host name")", before I leave I must tell the audience how to contact me. You may have to speak a little more quickly but speak as clearly as possible. While the host may have deliberately omitted giving you time to plug your business, this is very rare if you have done a good job. But whatever the reason, under no circumstances let the show end without plugging your business. Remember to keep your voice clear and calm even though you may be rushed, and try not to add any additional words. Let your contact information be the last words you speak, if at all possible.

Promotional Gifts

One way to entice listeners to contact your business is to offer them a gift or other giveaway. Many times guests will add a little fun for the listeners by letting them know that if they mention the station when they (call, visit the website, etc.) they will receive a percentage off the services, related materials or other gifts. I advise my nursing coach clients that are listed on my www.RNHealthCoach.com website, to use gimmicks sparingly, due to the nature of the profession. People take their health seriously and you may lose some credibility if the gimmicks or overdone. However, if you do choose to have listeners mention the radio show, the station will appreciate the boost in their ratings that will result. It is possible they will show their appreciation by booking you on other shows or giving you referrals for their sister stations.

Even if you don't participate in gifts and giveaways on a regular basis, you can use seasons and other events as special occasions to promote your business. For instance, you can offer discounts on smoking cessation coaching during a quit smoking month. Gifts to clients during the Christmas season or New Years weight loss discount coupons can also be a good idea. Since listeners will view you as an expert in your field, you can offer them a few health tips via email as a gift for signing up for your newsletter.

Gift and Promotional Ideas

If done properly, there is nothing wrong with offering potential clients a little gift incentive. Naturally, you don't want to cheapen the services you offer by giving away too much. But as we learned earlier in the book, greed and desire are strong motivators. So, you may reel in a long term client if you give them a free gift. This strategy has been used by many of my clients. Following the suggestions in this book, you can also run a giveaway campaign that will enhance your business.

Your website traffic is an essential element in the promotion and marketing of your business. That is why one of my services found at(www.MedicalMarketingSEO.com), utilizes the latest technology and experience to develop professional websites and optimize their content so that they are seen by millions. If you are interested in offering gifts to encourage viewers to select your services, my staff will include an email sign-up page where you can reward viewers for subscribing to your newsletter. To entice your website viewers, callers and other potential clients, the following are a couple of gifts or prizes you can offer for very little money.

-**Lists or charts.** Offer potential clients a list of information related to your nursing specialty. For instance, you can compile a "free" list of nursing coaches across the country based upon their need for services.

They can use this list if they live in another state or if they have a friend or relative living elsewhere who may need nurse coaching. You can also compile statistics on related medical matters; some clients will appreciate saving time researching their topic. Charts not only appeal to the logical side of the brain, they also provide an interesting visual option from lines of unbroken text. Make a few colorful pie charts or graphs and save them in a file. Offer them as giveaways or gifts to potential clients.

-**Free or low cost services.** I have touched on this one earlier. You can always offer a discount for new clients, seasonal discounts or free services as a gift during the holiday season.

-**Incentives to succeed.** You may want to promote that you will take a percentage of remaining coach sessions when a client reaches a certain milestone. For example, a percentage off the next weight loss session after ("x amount) of weight loss. Or, you can offer a gift or other incentive to clients that remain smoke free after a certain length of time.

-**Promotional materials.** Marketing materials such as pens, bookmarks and other small items are very inexpensive. You can offer to send a small thank you gift to people who make inquires or sign up for your newsletter. These serve as a nice little thank you and do double duty in spreading the word out about your company. Since they are so inexpensive, don't skimp on how they look. Make these as unique and eye catching as possible to draw attention to your business.

After the Show Etiquette

As the exit music plays, you will breathe a sigh of relief because you know you have completed your interview as planned. You stayed calm and professional and were an entertaining and engaging guest. Both you and your host are pleased with how it turned out and you've been told the phone lines are lit up with callers. However, your tasks are not complete just because the microphones have been turned off. After you've finished with your successful interview, there are a few things you should do to increase your chances of getting referrals and being invited back to the show.

At the end of the show the last words you should say is a thanks for being invited to the show. If you have completed a phone interview, stay on the line even after you realize the mike has been turned off. The producer will come back on the line to thank you and ask you any questions as needed. Do not forget this in the excitement because if you are not on the line they can view this as rudeness. During this after show conversation, it is appropriate to ask for a recommendation letter. If you can't request it during that time (for instance, if you and/or the producer are pressed for time), then just include the request in your follow up call or letter of thanks. Once you have completed these pleasantries, the interview is officially "a wrap" and you can hang up the phone and think about how the interview will greatly improve your business's exposure. Try not to immediately go into a mindset of critiquing everything you said or did during the interview. While constructive criticism can be helpful, give yourself a little time to bask in the success of what you have just accomplished. Pat yourself on the back for doing the best job you could. More than likely, you will be harder on yourself than is called for, and you will realize this once you get feedback from the producer and the host.

Don't Stop Now: Continuing Radio Marketing

I cannot stress how important it is for you to keep promoting your business. Even if you have several successful radio interviews under your belt, you still must continue to push for more. Marketing is a committed effort, and if you want your business to enjoy longevity, you must commit to years of marketing and promotion. You do not want to run the risk of your business falling off the radar screen. As you know, the competition will make sure that their name stays in view of the public.

Knowing this, don't slack off with your marketing, especially since you are getting free advertising through radio marketing. I have seen so many potentially great businesses fold because the owners did not keep up with advertising. This, in my opinion, is such a waste of time, energy and talent, especially when literally thousands of dollars in free advertising via radio interviews is so readily available. On the other hand, I have personally experienced the benefits of regular, consistent through marketing and promotion, including radio interviews.

Your most essential tool to stay on top of your promotion efforts will be my database. In order to keep fresh with your advertising efforts, you must keep an updated database because the radio business has a high turnover rate. My database is updated every six months, at a minimum. And I always come across a good number of stations with personnel changes each time I update. For you, this means that there will be new hosts and producers that you will need to pitch. You will also come across producers that have had you as a guest on another station in the past. You should make the rounds pitching to these producers as well since they are familiar with you, your work and what a good radio show guest you are. Most likely, you will run across a few who have lost your contact information and possibly have been looking for you when they changed radio stations. This networking option won't cost you a dime and can reap you many marketing benefits.

The bottom line is that non-stop promotion has to become a way of life for you in order for your business to remain successful. The good news is that you have tools, such as this book, that will guide you in your ongoing promotional efforts. Each of my businesses is also available to you for resources, help and support. I most certainly understand what you are going through each step of the way, and I will use my expert knowledge to help you enjoy success for your efforts.

Post Interview Success

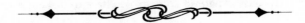

Repeat Interviews

I concluded the last chapter by encouraging you to never stop promoting your business. As I have throughout this book, I always try to follow up my suggestions by giving you practical advice on how to carry them out using radio interviews and several other means. I will begin this chapter by providing you with strategies to secure repeat interviews. Producers will invite you back for repeat interviews if you have employed the methods we have discussed throughout this book. Radio shows are very eager to have guests that are well prepared with interesting and insightful topics. They will remember and appreciate that, as a guest, you gave your full attention to the interview and were careful to be polite and respectful to the host and the audience. Sending that great thank you letter after the interview is sure to seal the deal. You will once again be asked to be a guest on the radio show. Here are a few pointers that will help you get repeat interviews.

- Unless the producer calls you sooner, wait about six months before pitching for a follow up interview. It is not your intention to annoy the producer by calling too soon.

- Try to have some new material or a different viewpoint on the same material ready before you are called or prior to you pitching for the new interview.

- If there is breaking news that is hot off the press that relates to your topic, you should make that call, even if less than six months has passed since the last interview.

- Remember, as a health care expert, there is no shortage of information that you can share with radio listeners. Capitalize on this by continually creating fresh content to be used for new or repeat interviews.

- One aspect of your repeat interview pitch can be to remind the producer of the great response from listeners at your last interview (if this was indeed the case). Promise to do your best to provide an even bigger response. If they book you based on this strategy, begin tweaking whatever content you have to make it even better.

- Here's a tip that I've given my clients that has resulted in more repeat interviews. When you are initially booked, have a chat with the producer about when he or she is next scheduled for vacation. Ask the producer if they will add your interview to the schedule of shows that will re-air doing their vacation time. You might even want to make it a habit of noting when the producer will be on vacation and take the initiative to ask just prior to the producer leaving.

Link to the Radio Station Website

Every radio station keeps a website up and running. It is common knowledge that a great website should have, among other features, interesting content. Without engaging content, visitors will quickly click off the page no matter how many polls, advertisements, games or other bells and whistles are incorporated in the site. Every business is always seeking relevant and fresh content to improve their website and draw more visitors. You can give your radio interview marketing some extra mileage by adding content that includes a link to your website.

While many websites, such as www.RNHealthCoach.com do have a page completely dedicated to links, you will be more successful with a radio website if you offer to post interesting content which will add value and incorporate your link within. All it takes is a little creativity to create an interesting article that ties in your nursing coach expertise with a topic that would be interesting to listeners and website visitors.

Then it's simply a matter of emailing this article to the webmaster or to the producer. Because your link is embedded in the article, your website will be networked in with the station's website, which, as you know, receives millions of hits each month.

Contact the producer, who may or may not refer you to the station's webmaster, to hammer out the details of this arrangement. Make sure that you are clear on the terms for posting your article.

For example, confirm whether you want to give permission for the webmaster to edit your content, whether they will expect fresh content on a regular basis, if they want a reciprocal link from your website, etc. In addition to getting even more free publicity, you will probably be invited back to the show as appreciation for your contribution to their site as well as get more exposure for a shot at new bookings.

Expand Your Reach

You will be successful at booking interviews because you are an expert in your field, with a wealth of information regarding health care. You do not have to limit your free marketing efforts to just radio, however. If you are contacted to speak by universities or other learning institutions, make time in your schedule to accommodate the request. In some instances, not only does this provide an opportunity to promote your business, but can also be a way for you to generate income.

Directories

Continue to promote your business by posting in magazines and directories. Several of these, including the Radio Television and Interview Report, let you advertise that you are interested in doing radio interviews. They will help you prepare a good pitch and post your pitch to their over 4,000 media producers that read the report.

Well Known Publications

I have helped business owners to promote their companies by featuring them in major publications. One way in which you can do this is to contact the publication directly with an article or story relating to your profession. Large magazines, both online and in print, will accept submissions of written material. Even national and international magazines, such as the New York Times, USA Today and Entrepreneur accept article submissions. With your nursing knowledge, you can promote your business by writing a story or article and sending it to magazines like Good Housekeeping, Women's World and others. There are also paid services that will offer subscriptions to receive email alerts when a publisher or editor is seeking material related to your field.

Television

When it comes to promoting your business, no media form is off limits. When you are ready, shoot for the stars and start looking for ways to market your business on television. Did you know that the aforementioned Radio Television Interview Report maintains a directory of the top television shows in the nation? There you can find all the contact information for shows such as Larry King, 20/20 and the 700 Club. National television news stations are also included in the directory such as CNN and Fox News. The database is very similar to my comprehensive database of top radio shows, where additional information about listeners and other demographics are included.

Many people who are looking to promote themselves take it to the next level by attending events such as the National Publicity Summit in New York. The summit is attended by some of the top television show producers in the country. While you can expect to pay to attend the summit plus the cost of travel, when you are ready, this will be an expense that will prove to be well worth it in the long run.

A Professional Website

Developing and maintaining a website is an absolute essential in today's age of technology. Your website will go a very long way in promoting you and what you do to the entire world. It is also a means to connect your business to your potential clients with a click of the mouse. Because of its importance, do not skimp on form or content when it comes to your website. Equally important, your website must be search engine optimized, so that when people scour the search engines looking for nursing coaches your website will be at the top of the list.

Even though you may be somewhat Internet savvy, the website for your business should be developed by a professional company. Although free interfaces are available that allow people to create their own site in just a few clicks, it is in your best interest to leave that for personal websites for entertainment or to connect with family. My marketing and promotion services have now expanded to offer a wide range of website development options by a team with years of experience and expertise. When you are ready to show off your business on the World Wide Web, visit my website at www.MedicalMarketingSEO.com for a list of services and costs.

The possibilities are endless for you to get the word out about your nursing coach practice. Thousands of people have seen their fledgling businesses grow into huge enterprises by advertising through various media. I am confident that you can also utilize the options I've outlined in this book to promote your nursing coach practice. I have shared the suggestions, ideas and information in this book based upon my own experience and knowledge of the nursing coach industry. Refer to the chapters within this book to refresh your memory or to help guide you along the way.

Many successful nursing coaches have led the way for you in utilizing this book and other resources to map out an individual plan for their success. Nothing will give me more joy than to hear your success stories and how using radio marketing and other media advertising has resulted in your personal and professional fulfillment. I hope to hear from you soon.

Conclusion

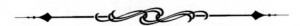

I sincerely thank you for taking the time to read this book. My hope is that it has proven to be a resource that you can use as a guide and reference, both now and in your future endeavors. I have written this book to encourage, inspire and equip you to make the most of your special gifts and talents that have enabled you to start your nursing coach practice.

As you work towards getting the word out about your business, never lose sight of the fact that as a registered nurse, you have the advantage over other wellness coaches. You have medical training that you can offer clients in areas of nutrition and diet, emotional wholeness and other in-depth medical training such as diagnosing health challenges. Remember to include these skills, training and education as you promote your business. Market as many of these skills as you possibly can, placing emphasis on the fact that you are extremely well rounded. Be sure to include your success stories, references and credentials when you are promoting your business. And don't forget to showcase your great personality and ability to work with all types of people during your promotional efforts.

As a marketing tool, the radio interview is invaluable for many reasons. In addition to it being a source of free advertising for you, it is a media that reaches millions of people from all walks of life. As you have learned from reading this book, it can be one of the best ways to promote your new business if executed properly. Even if you were to pay thousands of dollars for advertising via commercials, there is no guarantee that people will hear it. It has been proven that people often channel surf during radio commercials, much like the way they get up for a drink during television commercials. These are some of the inside "tricks of the trade" that you can use to boost your exposure.

If at any time you need support and assistance, my media outreach and public relations services are readily available for you. I assure you that I will use my many years of nursing experience, degree in business administration marketing and master's degree in finance to help you. I am able to give you my expert advice because of the comprehensive services in all aspects of the nursing coach business that I own that has helped so many others.

My umbrella company, L.I.T.E. Therapeutics, has for years worked tirelessly to network people with various health issues to independent nursing professionals. The company is the first (and only) to successfully tap into the unique talents of Registered Nurses and use those talents to support them in health coaching enterprises. This successful network includes a nationwide nurse coaching support, network and resource effort (www.RNHealthCoach.com) that offers these nursing entrepreneurs everything needed to succeed in their businesses. My organization has grown over the years to extend supportive services for these professionals to include promotion and marketing as well as website design and maintenance, including SEO services

How does all of this benefit you during this transition in your own career? I have experienced firsthand and mastered the steps you are now taking. Over the years, I have been on "both sides of the fence", so to speak, and have become an expert in the nursing industry in all aspects. I have gained extensive knowledge in caring for patients, medical conditions, diagnosis and treatment and the myriad of other nurse related skills. On the other side of the equation, I have personally gone through the process of developing and managing businesses, including promoting my businesses through several types of media. Therefore, the advice and suggestions that I share in this book are not simply from something I've read, but from my own actual experience. I have incorporated my experiences, education, research, success and even failures into a proven strategy that I know will work for you as well.

One example is the information I wrote in this book about hiring a public relations firm to promote your business. My own research and experience allowed me to give you practical advice about this option in order for you to make a decision that would work best for you. Having to juggle my own budget as I began this enterprise, I well know that a public relations firm can be a large expenditure. Most will request that you pay a non-refundable retainer and big monthly payments without a guarantee they will book interviews. I supplied you with examples of issues that you should watch for if you decide to hire a PR firm such as a firm that places emphasis on top markets and wattage. It is my hope that you can use practical tips such as these and adapt them to your own situation.

As you move forward with radio marketing, remember others who have been extremely successful in using this strategy. Let the stories of authors, celebrities and other business owners motivate you not to give up. Reflect on how many commercials you hear on any given day, and how many times you've purchased something based upon what you heard on a commercial. Translate this image into how many people you can reach over the radio and the awesome affect it can have on your business. And best of all, this can be accomplished at no cost to you!

You have learned how radio interviews are a win-win situation for both you and the radio station. Use this information to your advantage when attempting to book your interviews. Sell yourself as the expert that you are, keeping in mind that the media needs people with your kind of expertise in order to keep people listening. I explained to you the importance of combining this expertise with an entertaining and engaging style, a winning combination that is sure to get you booked for interviews. Please don't underestimate this as it can be the lethal weapon you use to jump ahead and stay ahead of your competition.

Leave no stone unturned when it comes to promoting your business. Use radio interviews to announce your services and to provide your phone number, website and other contact information. Never be ashamed of plugging your business, as each plug translates into potential clients and business growth. Brace yourself for a surge in inquires from potential clients each time you plug your business.

Throughout this book, I have crunched the numbers for you to provide statistics to underscore certain points related to advertising. Use these statistics to make wise decisions about how and where you will promote your business. Since two thirds of radio listeners tune in to an average of six radio stations every week, choose this media as the superior, free choice to start your advertising campaign. As I developed the marketing and promotion business (www.PRHealthCareCommunciations.com) I researched the times when people are more likely to listen to the radio in order to help my clients with scheduling their interviews. Early morning commuters make up a large percentage of listeners, but someone is listening in all times of the day, the fewest numbers being during the overnight hours. Close to eighty-five percent of people 12 and over in America tune in to the radio every day. Don't miss the opportunity to tap into this vast pool of potential clients.

I want to encourage you to employ the strategy of using statistics in your own business promotion. Most people trust and rely on statistics to support facts. And some people prefer to quickly read through statistics to form a conclusion rather than read a large amount of information. I have successfully used this in my own business promotion. I supply readers with health statistics that include numbers about the cost of health care and modifiable health risks, which is very interesting information.

You can adapt this method in your own coaching practice. For example, if your coaching will focus on smoking cessation, you can include demographic statistics related to smoking, smoking and gender as well as statistics on chances of quitting and staying smoke free in your promotional material. The same methods can be applied if weight loss and maintenance are your coaching specialty. And if it is overall wellness and health, you have a virtually limitless supply of research to draw from and to share in the form of statisticsRefer to the pages in this book often on your journey. As you are preparing for that first interview, refer to the wealth of information found in the chapter "Preparing for the Actual Interview". Start with getting organized and prepare an interview log so you can keep track of your bookings. Make the document so that you can quickly compile all information related to the booking including complete radio station, producer and host information. Although it may seem like a small detail, you need to indicate the format of the interview on the log, whether it will be taped or live, via telephone or in the studio.

It is imperative that you are consistent with this log because in the excitement you are bound to forget small details. In addition, the log can serve as a journal of sorts so that you can look back on it and see your progress.

I know firsthand the juggling act that it takes to schedule interviews once the ball gets rolling. Make sure you don't make the mistake of trying to schedule interviews without having your current schedule right in front of you. Among the practical tips I shared with you are the ideal days and times for radio interviews. Fridays are the least favorite because commuters who have listened to your show only have the one day to share what they heard before the weekend break. For morning shows, try to book that 7:30 to 8:30am time slot to snag those commuters caught in traffic with their radios tuned in.

If the radio producer shows interest in booking you, your call should always politely request, but not insist, on the premium spots. Booking about a week ahead leaves time for confirmation, advance promotion and for you to send any additional information that the station may request. But whatever time slot you are booked, keep up with current time zones at all cost. Remember to adjust for Daylight Savings Time and if you are on the east coast and happen to book an early morning show from the west coast, do not let the time zone difference show in your voice.

Not every radio station is the same. Size, location, format and audience are just some of the factors that set every studio apart from others. And not every interview will fall into identical categories. You must know the variations in stations and interviews long before you begin to pitch your business. Be prepared to tape live on the majority of your radio interviews. This means that you are being broadcast "in real time", so to speak.

One of the exceptions to this is interviews for music stations, which are usually taped in advance and aired when the station decides to do so. As you gain experience and courage, however, you will feel confident enough to convince even music stations that you are such an exciting, entertaining and professional expert that they need not worry about interviewing you live on the air. In the meantime, try to book as many live interviews as possible. Live interviews have the advantage of being heard by a potentially larger audience since you never know when a taped interview will be aired. Also, a live interview gives you experience with listener feedback and interaction.

Whether taped or live, I learned that there are some advantages and disadvantages to interviewing by phone and in the studio. Certainly, taping via telephone is very convenient. For one thing, you can reach listeners all over the entire country without having to travel. You can do phone interviews right in your own home, without having to be concerned with how to dress. And if you are somewhat shy, phone interviews can be a good way to get used to being interviewed.

Even so, studio interviews may be to your advantage in several ways if the studio is within a reasonable driving distance. Interviewing in the studio gives you the chance to meet with the producer in person, putting a face to the voice you've been hearing over the phone. You will also personally interact with the show host, which makes for a livelier interview as well as potential future bookings if all goes well. I have found that studio interviews tend to have a slight better sound quality. And I also appreciate being able to immediately get an audio copy of my interview at the studio when I bring a blank CD or pocket drive. I have also used studio interviews as an opportunity to network with sister stations that may occupy the same building as the studio in which I am interviewing.

For many reasons, studio interviews can be more advantageous to your promotion. However, there is one thing I want you to consider in conclusion of this issue. Whatever happens, do not let your preferences about the interview location, or any other issue, cause you to disrespect or insult the producer. Remember that the whole point in this marketing campaign is to build up your reputation as a professional and competent expert guest whom is easy to get along with. Make your requests known in a polite manner, but tune in to indications that the producer will not budge on the matter, and know when to give in if you have to.

Do not go to any type of interview unprepared. When you are booked for a phone interview, you have options to make the interview go as smoothly as possible. Make a connection with the station's operator before the interview, preferably the day before. This small interaction can pay off when calls for you come in after the interview. The operator will be sure to remember your friendliness and polite demeanor, which the operator will then pass on to your potential clients. This is also a good idea just in case there are some changes that need to be made on your contact information or a mistake in scheduling. Plan ahead for your phone interview by making sure the room where you will do the interview is neat, organized and isolated from any type of disturbances. Have your notes right near the phone, along with water and pen and paper. Of course, check and double check your alarm clock to make sure you wake up on time, which should be early enough for you to be fully awake when the interview begins.

I recommend even more preparation for my clients that are scheduled for in-studio interviews. To begin with, your appearance is of utmost important. This does not mean you have to dress formal enough to go to an inaugural ball. In fact, you are going to take your cues on how to dress from what you have seen the host wear. But since the show is on the radio, how do would you know how the host dresses? This is where advance preparation comes in. Take some time before your interview to go on the website of the radio station. There should be some photos of the host and other station employees that will give you a general idea about how to dress. But you basically cannot go wrong if you simply wear slacks or nice jeans and shirt if you are male, and slacks or a casual dress if you are a woman.

When you pack for the trip to the studio, make sure you bring a blank CD or drive so you can get a copy of the interview. Also, include extra copies of your information cards and a copy of the sample questions you prepared. Confirm directions, parking availability and studio security access before you leave, so you don't risk running late for the interview. The key point is to leave nothing to chance; don't let anything become a reason for you to end up feeling rushed or frustrated by the time the interview begins.

I spent years learning about the different types of radio stations and how these differences would affect my marketing strategies. Among the many things I did learn was how to differentiate between stations that will be useful to your efforts and those that might just be a waste of time. As you make your rounds doing interviews, there will be times when you will get an unsolicited call from stations that want to interview you.

Naturally, if it is a well-known station, you will know the call is a legitimate opportunity to promote your business and you wouldn't hesitate to accept the invitation. However, you will get calls from producers that you are unfamiliar with, so study the section called "When the Radio Show Contacts You" in the chapter entitled "Must Know Tips on Contacting Radio Shows and Booking the Interview".

This chapter goes into detail about the various types of stations as well as producers from less than legitimate shows. You will be reminded how to handle offers from very small stations and why you should be careful in doing so. Details about Internet radio shows, nationally syndicated shows and satellite radio are also covered in this chapter. If you've ever wondered, as I did when I first started, what are brokered radio shows, review this chapter to get some really insightful information about this topic.

When it comes to booking interviews, the bottom line is that it simply won't happen unless you have a terrific pitch. The pitch is your first (and sometimes last) shot at presenting your show idea, so it has to be well written, concise and well rehearsed. Your delivery of the pitch has to exude the confidence and professionalism that has led you to this point in your career. Don't make the mistake of pitching your individual business. I had to learn this for myself. What producers want to hear is an idea for their show, one that will entertain and inform their audience. Remember, your business will be promoted sometime during the course of the interview, but to get your foot in the door you must convince the producer that you have what it takes to make an interesting radio show, not a commercial. If not, rest assured you will be mistaken for someone who needs to speak with the paid advertising department of the radio station. The advice that I shared on this subject came from what I came to learn over years of experience in pitching my various businesses.

In all truthfulness, the conclusion of the matter is that none of the information in this book will be necessary if you don't have an absolutely first rate press kit. This is because the press kit is a hard copy representation of you and your business. With it, the producer will have no idea who you are, including your credentials and the vision of your businesses. The press kit can have so much impact and influence that I have personally seen bookings on huge radio stations based upon the press kit alone.

No matter how long it takes to compose, do not consider skipping this vital step in your marketing and promotion. I'm not saying that every person promoting their business has a press kit, but the ones that have the most impressive ones more often than not impress producers to want to see and hear more. Think of your press kit as the comprehensive, hard copy of your pitch. It will replace your physical presence in the boardroom when producers and hosts meet to brainstorm about ideas for radio shows.

If drafted to perfection or as closely as possible to perfection, your press kit makes a statement about your credibility and imagination. You have in your hands all of the information needed that should be included in an excellent press kit; starting with the portfolio the kit should be housed in, down to the details to be included in your biography, photograph and contact information. I am confident that if you use this book as a guideline, you will know the exact specifications that producers find impressive in a press kit.

The press kits that I utilize for my businesses are carefully planned and organized. I accept no less than the highest level of professionalism with my press kits since I am very aware of their importance. I give producers an idea of my personality by briefly describing why I started my business enterprises. My biography (yours should always be included in your kit) includes my photograph, in my uniform, to paint a picture of the pride I have in my profession. The verbiage in my biography exudes the confidence I have without sounding boastful. For instance, I include in my press kit that I am a visionary whose ideas led me to the development of my umbrella company, L.I.T.E. Therapeutics, Inc. I mention that I coined the title of my nursing coach networking organization found on my website www.RNHealthCoach.com. Highlighting the fact that you are creative in your press kit is one of the ways that you can convey to the producers that you have the potential to be a creative and flexible radio show guest.

In each of my press kits, I am sure to include my credentials. This includes my education, nursing experience and any media experience that I have. You too, should let your press kit describe your background and experience. Include the length of time so that the producer gets an idea of your longevity. And don't leave out any past and current professional organizations to which you belong. As an example, my press kits include the fact that I am a member of several organizations including the American Heart Association and the American Diabetes Association. This information also helps producers to get a sense of the commitment you have to your profession and your desire to remain current on the latest nursing and health news.

Never stop looking for show ideas to use for your pitch. We are in a profession that is ideally suited for innumerable topics that make for great show ideas. Health care, in one fashion or another, is on the minds of just about every citizen in the country. It is your ongoing task to find ways to tie in this interest in health care in a way that will stimulate the minds of listeners. Your show ideas can stem from the latest headlines that may not scream health care, but will no doubt relate to a health care issue.

Take, for example, the state of the economy that is discussed in print media, television and radio on a daily basis. Have you ever thought of the effects on the physical and mental health of people who are struggling to make ends meet in this economy? Or, would the stress of paying bills cause people to either start or relapse in their addictive behaviors such as cigarette smoking? And how about what this economy has done as it relates to finding employment as a nurse? I have sometimes used this take on nursing and the economy in my press kits. In fact, the beginnings of my idea for developing a nursing coach network began with my desire to help nurses who were not able to find employment. By tying in the need for nurses to become financially independent with the desire of consumers to be proactive in their own health, I was able to develop a unique and interesting concept.

Make brainstorming for show ideas a scheduled task each week. As I advised you in this book, keep current on all news events and watch for those that relate to your specialty. Other ideas for shows can be experiences you may have had in your personal life. Success stories you've enjoyed with your clients also make for inspiration and entertaining shows that producers will appreciate and audience will tune in to.

No matter how practiced, educated and talented we are, in the end we are all just human beings. That is why I felt it important to include extensive information about emotions and how they affect you, the host and the audience. As professionals and business owners, part of our natural character is to assert ourselves and our viewpoints. But, as we learned, such assertion must be tempered with self control when it comes to a radio interview. You learned how certain points in an interview must be conveyed before the end of the interview, or it does not serve to promote your business. You cannot take a doormat stance, shyly and passively allowing a host to take total control without getting your key messages across to the audience. Remain focused on your sole purpose for agreeing to the interview and by all means have the confidence to assert yourself if you have to.

I am not trying to give you the impression that every show host will try to cheat you out of promoting your business because this is not the case. In fact, the majority of hosts are more than happy to turn over the flow of the show to you, if you show that you are capable of doing so. It takes practice to know how to do this without appearing to bully your host or the audience but trust me; it can be done.

It was equally important for me to share with you what I've learned about the emotions of the audience. People are motivated to tune in to radio shows that feature experts on various subjects for many reasons. In the case of our profession, fear of illness, disease or even death may be the reason a person tunes in to hear our interview. In fact, fear is the strongest of all human emotions. Greed is another strong emotion that may prompt a listener, or maybe they feel they can get free medical or other advice. Anger, as you know is a powder keg emotion that can explode in a negative way if not controlled. Some people tune in and call radio shows for no other purpose than to vent a seething anger. In some cases, the anger may be justified, such as the mistreatment of children or elderly. But as unfortunate as it may be, sometimes people are just plain angry about an experience in their own lives and will use a call to your show as the target upon which to vent this anger.

This is why the section on how to handle audience calls had to be written. When you are on an interview that will invite audience participation, be prepared to meet the challenges that will undoubtedly follow. Now, not all of these challenges will be negative. For instance, you may get a call of thanks for sharing your information, or you may be asked a question that you can answer so insightfully that it makes you look good. By far, these are the majority of calls that will come in.

However, radio stations routinely screen incoming calls before putting the caller on the air, and for very good reasons. As I mentioned, a call that you know is meant to hurt, disparage or undermine your credibility may sneak by and you will want to immediately lash out at the caller. But don't jump the gun and verbally retaliate. If they have a question and it is a valid one, try to answer it as calmly as possible, no matter how it was delivered. But, rather than risk losing the respect of the listening audience, save the retorts and verbal assaults. This does not mean that you should allow yourself to be abused and misrepresented. You can and should defend yourself against deliberate attacks. One way I have learned to handle such situations is to take notice of how my host interacts with the caller and then follow his or her lead.

Along the same lines, you must master your emotions when it comes to dealing with the radio show host. Gracious, charming and professional show hosts are the norm in the industry. But despite this fact, there are some hosts that will simply rub you the wrong way. You can never, I repeat never, allow your demeanor to reveal that you find any host to be egotistical or snobbish. Even if you realize that the agenda of the host is to spark a debate to increase audience interest, don't let this bait you into a viewing it as a personal battle. Instead, take this as exactly what it is: a part of being in show business. At the show's end, politely thank your host and put the rest out of your mind.

Take some time periodically to brush up on all of the strategies you have learned in this book. Study the fine points of preparing for an actual interview. You will need to know how to handle delays or rescheduling of an interview and the reasons that they occur. Master communication techniques and show business etiquette so that you come off as a polished and professional expert. Even if you tend to be the nervous type, study and practice can greatly help with any insecurity you may have about live broadcasting. Stretch your ability to adapt to different circumstance and people. Use this book to show you how to be flexible when it comes to speaking the language of your audience.

Like many others before you, there is a need to face the challenge of focusing on the main points you want to get across during an interview. In the excitement of the moment, even the most seasoned interviewees can go completely off track about why they are there. With practice and determination, you can learn to streamline your notes so that they become a reflection of the bullet points in your press kit. That way, you are sure to pull yourself together and hit the key notes should you become distracted during the interview.

As I've said to you before, you will reach the point when the first interview is behind you. As you've learned, this is not the time to take a break. You need to become an expert in effective follow up with the station, producer and host. You need to know how to impress the producer to the point that you are irresistible and sure to be called back for a follow up interview. Let this book be your resource during all of the exciting stages of your business marketing and promotion, for that is what it is intended to be.

I wrote this book to motivate you to reach optimal levels of success in your private nursing coach practice. Throughout the book, I have attempted to convey to you that you do have support before, during and after this exciting venture. My desire was also to inform you of the many tools in which I have become expert in using that have led to the expansion of my company in the public relations services and media outreach industries. These same tools were vital in my success as an RN, author, visionary and CEO of several companies. As you read this book, you may have wondered why I included certain topics and not others. Actually, I believe I have shared with you in this book information on topics that were of great benefit to me throughout my journey. My hope is that I will continue to share with you new information as I learn long into the future.

In my opinion, the only definite conclusion that can be reached regarding radio marketing is that there is no conclusion. Because, take it from me, just when you think you have mastered one aspect of the business, something new will come along and remind you how much there is to learn. In addition, you will have the constant knowledge that your competitors are hot on your track trying to obtain business that is meant for you.

I am certain that you feel as I do about your career and your business. There is never enough you can do to keep them healthy and viable. Whatever it takes - continuing education, non-stop promotions or 24 hour a day research - you have committed to support your vision and talent. This is the essence of marketing and promotion. Once you set foot on its path, you begin the rewarding and never-ending journey to fulfillment and the satisfaction of helping others that you have always dreamed of. I have no doubt you are up to the task.

About the Author

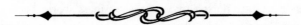

While Dwayne Adams has been an active and successful registered nurse for over a decade, working in critical care and emergency settings, he is also an accomplished entrepreneur. Capitalizing on his nursing expertise, he combined it with his business skills to create a successful new enterprise.

Along with his nursing education, Adams earned a bachelor's degree in business administration in the area of marketing, as well as a master's degree in finance. This education outside of the nursing field has given him the added edge he needed in order to become a successful entrepreneur and lead his company from growth through expansion.

His first business-related endeavor was to bridge the gap between registered nurses and those who could benefit from working with a health and wellness coach. With this idea in mind, he created a whole new concept and coined the term *"RN Health Coach."* His business concept of registered nurses becoming health coaches has been well received, and many nurses around the country have followed his lead and benefited from his advice.

As a business-savvy registered nurse, Adams not only created a lucrative new career field for those in nursing, but has also used his skills, education and experience to help them become successful entrepreneurs. He understands what it takes to build a business, market it, and sustain it long-term.

Given the state of health that people across the nation are currently in, Adams has shown his genius by creating the RN Heath Coach field. His passion for helping nurses to put their skills and education to use beyond the setting of a hospital bedside, combined with his entrepreneurial mindset, has created a lucrative field for registered nurses to enter.

He has developed a recipe for success that creates a win-win situation for all involved. Registered nurses get the pleasure of doing what they love – helping people – while those in the community who need health and wellness coaching get the most qualified coaches available.

Adams has a unique perspective on the business world because of his nursing background. This allows him to actively pinpoint the most effective ways for RN Health Coaches to build, promote, and enjoy their new career field. He is an expert in the areas of nursing and health and wellness coaching, but also in marketing, finance, and business

Other Titles

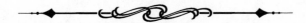

The Nurse Expert vol. 1, Secrets to being your own publicist.
ISBN: 978-0-9850033-1-9

The Nurse Expert vol. 2, How to use radio to position yourself as the authority in your field.
ISBN: 978-0-9850033-0-2

The Nurse Expert vol. 3, Your 3 Step formula for success.
ISBN: 978-0-9850033-2-6

Beyond The Bedside, Alternative Careers for Nurses.
ISBN: 978-0-9850033-3-3

Resource Websites

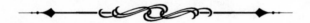

www.RNHealthCoach.com

www.HealthCoachNursingJobs.com

www.PRHealthCareCommunications.com

www.MedicalMarketingSEO.com

www.TheNurseExpert.com

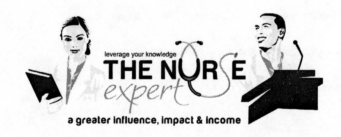

leverage your knowledge

THE NURSE
expert

a greater influence, impact & income

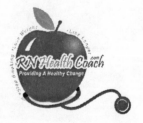